Dieting Makes You Fat

GEOFFREY CANNON and HETTY EINZIG

A guide to energy, food, fitness and health

SPHERE BOOKS LIMITED
London and Sydney

First published in Great Britain by Century Publishing Co. Ltd 1983
Copyright © Geoffrey Cannon and Hetty Einzig 1983
Revised, updated and expanded edition
published by Sphere Books Ltd 1984
30–32 Gray's Inn Road, London WC1X 8JL
Reprinted 1984 (three times)

TRADE
MARK

Set in 10/11pt Garamond

Printed and bound in Great Britain by
Collins, Glasgow

Geoffrey Cannon read Philosophy, Psychology and Physiology while at Balliol College, Oxford, and was a founder member of New Society. After ten years at the BBC, as Editor of Radio Times, he joined the Sunday Times in 1980 as Assistant Editor. In 1982 he devised the 'Getting in Shape' project, designed to investigate the relationship between fitness and health. He has also devised exercise programmes for Running magazine, for which he writes a monthly column. Geoffrey Cannon is now editor of New Health magazine.

Hetty Einzig is a freelance journalist whose interest in women's health and related issues began while studying Modern Languages at Girton College, Cambridge. She has written for the Sunday Times, Harpers & Queen and various other publications.

Geoffrey Cannon read Philosophy, Psychology and Physiology while at Balliol College, Oxford, and became a founder member of the Society.

After ten years at the B.B.C. as Editor of Radio Times, he joined the Sunday Times in 1980 as an editor and writer. In 1982 he devised the 'Getting in Shape' project, designed to investigate the relationship between fitness and health. He has devised exercise programmes for Running magazine, for which he writes a monthly column. Geoffrey Cannon is now editor of New Health magazine.

Hetty Einzig is a freelance journalist whose interest in women's health and related issues began while studying Modern Languages at Girton College, Cambridge. She has written for the Sunday Times, Harpers & Queen and various

ετον ετελιο καλαμαρα
και καλαμαρακια

and in memory of
Surgeon – Captain T L Cleave
1906 – 1983

Preface

This is not a diet book. It is a book about dieting. It is also a guide to energy, food, fitness and health.

By 'diet' and 'dieting' we are not referring to the quality of what people eat, because of their habits, beliefs or desire for health (as in 'vegetarian diet'). We are referring to the quantity, or rather lack of quantity, of food eaten, because of a desire to lose weight (as in 'calorie-controlled diet'). When we say that dieting makes you fat, we are using the word 'diet' in the sense of diet regime.

This book is not for people who are very fat indeed, who may, unfortunately, be suffering from a metabolic disorder and need special hospital treatment. A woman of normal height weighing, say, eighteen stone, or more, may need to be semi-starved and kept under medical supervision in order to regain health. We are writing for people who are not ill; for the scores of millions of people in the West who are fatter than they want to be, who have tried dieting, who have found that dieting does not work, and who want to know why.

We do not recommend the use of drugs as a means to lose weight. It is our conviction, shared by doctors who have supported us in the preparation of this book, that now is the time for people in the West to take responsibility for their own health and to avoid drugs whenever possible. Able-bodied people do not need drugs to lose weight, and any drug devised to suppress appetite or to speed up metabolism is liable to be as damaging to health as is nicotine and the other poisons in cigarettes.

The research for this book has been the joint responsibility of the two authors. The book has been written by Geoffrey Cannon, and the 'I' throughout the book is therefore his; with the exception of chapters 6 and 7, which are written from a woman's view by Hetty Einzig.

Acknowledgements

Professor Per-Olof Åstrand, Sir Douglas Black, Dr Denis Burkitt, Dr Kenneth Cooper, Dr Denis Craddock, Professor John Durnin, Dr Katherine Elliott, Dr Elizabeth Ferris, Dr John Garrow, Dr Kenneth Heaton, Dr Hugh Trowell, Caroline Walker and Professor Peter Wood read this book, or pertinent sections of it, before its hardback or paperback publication, gave us encouragement, and advice which we have incorporated.

Dr Keith Ball, Professor Michael Berger, Dr David Booth, Ben Cannon, Will Chapman, Dr Michael Church, Helen Cleave, Surgeon-Captain Hugh Cleave, Surgeon-Commander Brian Cliff, Dr Michael Colgan, Professor Michael Crawford, Dr Alan Maryon Davis, Mike Down, Wendy Doyle, Professor Richard Edwards, Susan Einzig, Malcolm Emery, Dr Oliver Gillie, Professor William Haskell, Professor Mark Hegsted, Victoria Huxley, Professor Philip James, Professor Harry Keen, William Laing, Dr Derrick Lonsdale, John McCarthy, Alistair Mackie, Mary Mackintosh, Tom McNab, Dr Michael Marmot, Professor J.N. Morris, David Nabarro, Dr Eric Newsholme, Professor Ralph Paffenbarger, Vic Ramsey, Dr John Rivers, Christopher Robbins, Dr David Ryde, Professor Bengt Saltin, Lillian Schofield, Professor Aubrey Sheiham, Dr Andrew Strigner, Professor Albert Stunkard, Professor Paul Thompson, Colin Tudge, Dr Richard Turner, Professor Arvid Wretlind, Brian Wright, Celia Wright, Arthur Wynn, Margaret Wynn, Dr John Yudkin and Professor John Yudkin gave us advice or guidance on particular aspects of the book.

We owe thanks to everyone who helped us. The responsibility for the views in the book is of course ours.

Once again, we will be glad to hear from any reader who wishes to comment on any points we make.

The climate that has allowed us to prepare the book has been created by friends, colleagues, and workers in the field, who we would also like to acknowledge.

At *The Sunday Times*, John Lovesey and Norman Harris have championed the cause of health and fitness for all; and Don Berry has supported our ideas. At *Running* magazine, Sylvester Stein, Alison Turnbull, and especially Andy Etchells, have supported the projects that turned some of the thinking behind the book into living experience. Cardiologists Dr Robin Hedworth-Whitty and Dr Peter Williams, together with physiologists Ted Charlesworth and Kevin Sykes, and Dick Hubbard, Rita Rowe and Ian Jamieson, supported these projects. At the Bodyworkshop Barbara Dale, Catherine Mackwood and Esme Newton-Dunn have shared their experience and enthusiasm.

For the *London 1982/50* project, special thanks are due to Will Chapman, Jim Cockburn, Rosemary Evison, John Goody, Joyce Goody, Michael Jacob, Hilda Nyman, Rosemary Tempest, and John Walker; to Terry Bennett, Peter Bird, Don Clark, Steven Downes, James Kelly, Ken Walker and Stan Weber; and above all to Simon Morris. For the *Fun Runner '82* project, as well as those already mentioned, special thanks are due to Bill Brown, James Godber, Dr Barrie Gunter, Mick Rankin, Bernie Tuck and Wendy Wood; and to Allan Appleton, Vic Burrowes, Tim Burton, Vivienne Coady, Bill East, Jane Heywood, Michael Innes, Rodney Lewis, Teresa Malinowska, Liz Parry, Bobbie Randall, John Routledge and Eileen Ward. For the *Getting in Shape* project, special thanks are due to Professor David Denison, Malcolm Emery, Dr Bob Green, Jane Howarth, Tom McNab, Dr Andy Peacock, Bev Risman, and the staff at the National Heart and Chest Hospital and the West London Institute; and above all to Will Chapman. Everyone connected with these projects is to be thanked; some three times over.

Personal support was given by Kathy Crilley, Corinne McLuhan, Teri McLuhan, Charlotte Parry-Crooke, Rosalind Schwartz, and by our families.

Sir Douglas Black, President of the Royal College of

Physicians of London, has been the presiding genius of three reports, on Medical Aspects of Dietary Fibre, Inequalities in Health, and Obesity, all of which have influenced us. Inspiration and encouragement has also been given by Graham Alexander, Dr June Burger, Dr Michael Cohen, Helen Davis, Bob Donovan, John Falkiner, Tim Gallwey, John Gravelle, Bob Kriegel, Ian McGarry, Michael Murphy, John Poppy, John Ridgway, Mark Shapiro, Paul Spangler, Leslie Watson and Sir John Whitmore, all of whom have contributed some spirit to the book.

Professor Marshall McLuhan became a dear friend and a teacher who encouraged the knowledge that progress often requires looking a paradox in the eye. This book is the poorer for having been written after his death.

Deborah Rogers, our agent, and Gail Rebuck, our publisher, together with Susan Lamb, Sarah Wallace and Anthony Cheetham, had the courage of our conviction. Penny Phipps and Deborah Brain put the show on the road. We owe special thanks to them.

Additional note

As the much longer list of acknowledgements in this new (paperback) edition indicates, we have been given the most generous encouragement, criticism and advice from authorities in Britain, Europe and America who, with us, are convinced that plenty of whole food and plenty of fresh air are not only the reliable treatment for overweight, but also the means to a full, happy and long life. Thanks to this support we have been able to incorporate much new research and new thought, together with other work we had overlooked, into this edition.

Above all we owe thanks to the hundreds of readers who have written to us, giving accounts of their own experiences and asking for advice. While we have not written a cook-book or a series of exercise programmes, we have, in response to readers, written new passages designed as practical guides to nutrition and exercise. So, this new edition is indeed 'revised, updated and expanded'.

Contents

Contents

Introduction

In January 1983 the Royal College of Physicians of London published a report on obesity. Commenting on surveys of British men and women in the last fifty years the report states: 'There now seems little doubt that there is a general trend for both men and women to become heavier and presumably fatter, this change being particularly evident in young adults'.

In common with the citizens of the USA and other Western countries, British people are getting fatter. In 1981, it was officially estimated that about a quarter of men and women in their twenties and just under half the population over forty are carrying excess weight. If you assume that these figures merely demonstrate that we are eating more, they will not surprise you. But we are eating less. British government statistics show that since 1960 we have consumed a steadily decreasing amount of energy from food and drink.

It is generally assumed that fat people are greedy and, certainly, that they not only eat too much but also more than lean people. How could it be otherwise? But in 1982 Alison Paul, a leading nutritionist, reported that British children and teenagers are eating less than their parents, are consuming anything from 300 to 500 calories a day less than World Health Organisation recommendations, yet are more likely to be overweight than underweight. Professor Harry Keen of Guy's Hospital conducted a survey of 3000 adults which showed that those who ate most had least body fat. And in 1983 Professor Peter Wood of Stanford University in California, reporting on studies carried out in Britain, the USA and other Western countries, said 'Generally speaking, fatter people eat less than thinner people.'

Diets slow you down

These facts are not well known simply because they are so puzzling. I have yet to read them in any diet book. This is no surprise, because they suggest what millions of dieters have found out for themselves: that diets do not work.

An older generation used to say that fat people were unlucky, because they had 'something wrong with their glands'. A more sophisticated version used the word 'genes' rather than 'glands'. A theory which went the rounds recently is that fat people are stuck with a 'set-point' programmed to make them fat. This is a variation of an older idea, that fat people are lumbered with a 'low metabolism'. From the point of view of the fat person who wants to be thin, all these theories are bad news. They all imply that there is not much anybody can do about being fat; that some people are born to be thin, others born to be fat, and, well, there it is.

But these notions cannot be right for one reason alone: the example of non-Western societies. People living in settled rural communities untouched by Western influence often live to a ripe old age and eat well without becoming overweight, let alone obese. Moreover, before the Industrial Revolution few people other than the rich in Western countries became fat. The theory that, all of a sudden, fatness became inherited, is absurd.

Every book on dieting tells you to concentrate on reducing the amount of energy you take in from food. And most will tell you that, while exercise is good for you, it won't make much difference to your weight. Stay sedentary but go on a diet, is the message. Yet recent studies have shown that active people are leaner and lighter than sedentary people, and lose weight as a result of exercise. And, also, active people eat much more food than sedentary people.

When we talk of 'metabolism' or, more correctly, 'metabolic rate' we are referring to the speed at which the body uses energy. The diet books assume that while different people have different metabolic rates, every individual has a fixed rate. That is to say, we are taught that we are stuck with the metabolic rate we are born with. And dieters are also led to believe that most, if not all weight lost on a diet, is fat. But scientists have known for more than fifty years that dieting slows the body down and certain types of exercise speed it up: well established facts that, if published in diet books, would damage their sales.

This was the point at which Hetty Einzig and I began the research for this book. And we came to realise that, much more often than not, dieting creates the conditions it is meant to cure. That is to say, dieting makes you fat.

Some diet books claim that their regimes can make you lose ten pounds or more in a week. This claim is accurate. But the weight lost is not fat. Nor is it merely water. It is also glycogen, a form of glucose stored in the muscles and liver, which is the immediately available energy needed by the body and brain. Loss of glycogen triggers intense sensations of hunger. Once a diet regime is ended the glycogen will be replaced. Have you ever read that in a diet book?

Exercise speeds you up

The exciting news is that metabolic rate is not static: it is dynamic. Within wide limits we can choose the speed at which we want our bodies to work, and we can gain a faster metabolic rate by the right kind of exercise. The body gradually adapts to endurance exercise by losing fat and gaining lean tissue. This training effect allows us to eat more while losing fat, because working muscle is very much more metabolically active than body fat.

It is only in the past few years, as a result of the running and aerobics boom in the USA, Great Britain and other Western countries, that millions of people have changed from being overweight dieters, to leaner, lighter, fit and healthy people, who exercise a lot and eat a lot too.

Diet books tell us to worry about the quantity of the food we eat, on the assumption that the basic requirement of the body is energy from food. This assumption is wrong too. The basic requirement of the body is not for quantity but for quality. What is wrong with the food we eat is its lack of quality; what the body needs is not so much energy as nourishment.

Good food – the recipe for health

The main single cause of the diseases that most of us in the West suffer and die from is the food we eat, together with inactivity. 'Western' diseases are typically of the heart and blood vessels (the cardiovascular system) and of the stomach and gut (the alimentary tract). Western food lacks nourishment because most of it is processed. Of all the processed foods we eat, sugar is unique in having no nourishment whatever.

Sedentary dieters, who eat least food of all, lead an unhealthy life; they cannot eat enough nourishing food even if they avoid processed food totally. Sedentary people who do eat enough nourishing food will become fat, simply because the only way they can get enough nourishment from food is to consume too much energy.

The sure way to good health is through fitness. Regular vigorous exercise gives the body the capacity for food for which it was designed. Regular exercise brings with it the freedom to eat as much as you like. Active people can best enjoy their lives by eating whole food, full of nourishment.

The best medicine is plenty of fresh air and plenty of good food: a remedy many family doctors once recommended, now obscured by big business, technology, drugs and surgery.

It is our conviction that dieting is not only self-defeating but also a means whereby tens of millions of men, and at least twice as many women, are prevented from enjoying their own lives.

You can change your life only when you know that you are able to make the change. Dieters often feel helpless not only about their weight and shape but about their lives; because they do not know how to become the shape and weight that is right for them. This book may encourage you to take your life back into your own hands.

CHAPTER ONE

Confessions of a Dieter

A man or woman may live and work and maintain bodily
equilibrium on either a higher or lower energy level. One
essential question is, what level is most advantageous? The
answer to this must be sought not only in metabolism
experiments and dietary studies, but also in broader
observations regarding bodily and mental efficiency and
general health, strength and welfare.

W O ATWATER AND F G BENEDICT
Bulletin of the US Department of Agriculture, 1902

Quality. You know what it is, yet you don't know what it
is. But that's self-contradictory. But some things *are* better
than others, that is, they have more quality. But when you
try to say what the quality is, apart from the things that
have it, it all goes poof! . . . Obviously some things are
better than others, but what's the *betterness*?

ROBERT C PIRSIG
Zen and the Art of Motorcycle Maintenance

Memoirs of a failed dieter

I found a slip of paper recently, folded into an old wallet.
It read:

    2 eggs boiled or poached
    4 ounces of lean meat OR boiled fish
    1 slice bread
    2 water biscuits
    ½ ounce butter (level dessert spoon)
    ½ ounce sugar (level dessert spoon)
    1 ounce milk (two coffees white)
    2 ounces hard cheese

in any amount:
water (three pints at least)
tea, coffee
gherkins, dry spices
peppers (only 'fruit' allowed)
lemon
chemical sweeteners
green salad (only vegetables allowed)

all else forbidden, including:
butter + ½ ounce
sugar + ½ ounce
alcohol
fruit, fruit juice

Dieting connoisseurs will recognise this daily regime as a version of the high-protein diets set out in *The Doctor's Quick Weight Loss Diet* by Dr Irwin Stillman and in *The Complete Scarsdale Medical Diet* by the late Dr Herman Tarnower. My version was sterner about fruit and vegetables, and cheated a bit with the butter and sugar.

Dr Stillman and Dr Tarnower disagree in some respects. But a lot of people believe in their diet regimes; to date, their books have sold a total of twenty million copies, world-wide. 'I'm convinced that the Quick Weight Loss Diet is the finest and best for most people who should take off excess weight,' wrote Dr Stillman in 1967. 'No diet has ever been as spontaneously and unanimously acclaimed as this one,' wrote Dr Tarnower in 1978. He went further: 'I urge you to get started now on this diet. Every day that you delay and keep or increase that extra poundage is impairing your appearance and your health, and is endangering and shortening your life. Overweight is a kind of death for almost everyone, slow for some, quicker for others.' Fervent words.

Weight lost – and regained

I first tried the high-protein diet in 1970. It worked. My weight came down by forty-one pounds, from thirteen stone eight pounds to ten stone nine, in twelve weeks. I had reached and passed my target.

In 1974 I went on the high-protein diet again. This time I followed the word of Stillman more faithfully, adding fruit, vegetables, tuna with all the oil drained, diet soda, and mustard to the regime. I cut out sugar and butter but allowed myself one sin – a glass of wine. It worked again. This time my weight came down from twelve stone twelve pounds by ten pounds in two weeks; by twenty pounds in four weeks; then the rate of loss slowed so that after six weeks I had lost twenty-five pounds. Then, after nine weeks, by a dizzying and ecstatic effort of will I broke the 150-pound barrier; and held steady at ten stone six pounds between weeks twelve and sixteen.

Like psychiatrists and schoolteachers, diet doctors often have a way of suggesting that if all goes according to plan the credit is theirs, whereas if you fail the fault is yours. I believed them. I had regained over thirty pounds between 1970 and 1974, despite two intermediate purges each of twelve pounds. And, by New Year's Day 1976, I had regained thirty-two pounds. At midnight I made a New Year resolution and, for a week, followed the regime set down in Dr Allan Cott's *The Ultimate Diet* and in Shirley Ross' *The Super Diet*. I fasted. Not a pea. Just water. Well, a small sin: milk in coffee.

After three days, I found, as the books said, that hunger faded, and I felt clean, light-headed and sharpened. More to the point, after ten days I had lost fifteen pounds, finishing up at eleven stone nine pounds. But, by the end of April, I had regained sixteen pounds.

My biggest weight loss was on a 'single-food' diet. These diets, often touted as fun, do not count calories but restrict the dieter to one (or a few) foods. The more ingenious versions stipulate a food normally seen as a treat, which, in due course, you come to hate. Examples are the grapefruit diet, the milk and banana diet and the ice-cream diet. Single-food diets are usually sold along with some mumbo-jumbo about the special qualities of the food to be eaten.

Judy Mazel's 'Beverly Hills Diet' is a skilfully marketed version of the single-food diet. It restricts the dieter to exotic fruits (mango, papaya, with pineapple) for days at a time. Since the average-sized woman would have to eat

3

eight pounds of mangoes a day to supply her normal energy requirement, it is hardly surprising that the Beverly Hills Diet works.

Ten-potato diet

Any single-food diet will work, whatever the food. In a classic experiment – of rather more nutritional significance than Ms Mazel's diet – twenty-three young Irishmen from Galway, organised by Dr Denis Burkitt, volunteered to eat ten large potatoes baked in their skins every day for three months. Most of them lost weight, for the potatoes represented about 1250 calories a day, less energy than the male body normally needs for its maintenance. No one yet has become rich and famous propagating this Irish diet, which is surprising in a way, since the volunteers were told that they could eat anything they liked every day, after they had eaten the potatoes. In the event they found they had little room left for pork chops or profiteroles.

My own version of the single-food diet was oranges – with the occasional tomato. The principle of this regime was that I liked oranges and tomatoes; and still do, surprisingly enough. In three months in 1967 I dropped over forty pounds, from thirteen stone three pounds to ten stone four. I celebrated by buying a suit, which fitted me for two days and which still hangs in my wardrobe, a memento of two days in my life when I was thin.

I was good at dieting. I could always win a lose-weight contest. My first epic diet was of the 'sensible' type recommended by Professor John Yudkin in his book *This Slimming Business* and, more recently, by the Consumers' Association in *Which? Way to Slim*: low carbohydrates; cut down, or out, bread, pasta, cereals, confectionery, cakes, biscuits, potatoes and alcohol. 'A low-carbohydrate diet is good for general health, not only for slimming,' says the *Which?* guide. This worked too: I lost over twenty pounds, which I regained in two years. It was, as I recall, this failure that led me to try most other diets, once. Nevertheless, on two or three other occasions I cut out the carbohydrates, regarding bread and potatoes, with sweets, as bad, and would lose seven to ten pounds in two or three weeks.

Between 1964 and 1976 I lost about 200 pounds. If all my diets had worked, on New Year's Day 1976 I would have weighed minus twenty pounds. But the records I kept were full of notes like 'half-way there!' and then 'failed' and 'failed again'. Most of my life consisted of backsliding from diets. Was it the spoon of sugar, the glass of wine? I supposed that between diet regimes I 'let go'; I felt bound to agree with Professor Yudkin:

> The upshot is that if you take too much food, containing too much fat and carbohydrate (or to a much lesser extent too much protein) you will be piling up an excess which you will store as fat . . . In the end, it is food, and only food, that makes you overweight.

I read this as meaning that I was greedy. Gaining weight was a visible sign of an inward weakness; of a general failure as a person. If I didn't diet I feared and believed that I would balloon up and become like the Michelin Man. These horrid fantasies drove me to diet regimes. Dieting is a private matter. Like 'dirty' books, diet books are not read in public places, because in both cases people are ashamed to reveal how they fall short of what is expected of them and what they want to expect of themselves. The best-selling British paperback of 1982 was Audrey Eyton's *The F-Plan Diet*, recommending fibre as a means to slim, which to date has sold over two million copies and has sold faster than any other British paperback except *Lady Chatterley's Lover*. But when I was a dieter in the 1970s I thought I was alone with my problems.

Trying psychology

I tried psychology. On another slip of paper I wrote 'Being Fat Means':

> Clothes don't fit. Good clothes hang, wasted, in the wardrobe. I pretend drab and baggy clothes are best.

> I get tired, especially at weekends. I loll around listlessly, and may even sleep in the afternoons.

Food is obsessive. I eat, feel bloated, and then feel hungry again. I look for eating companions.

Embarrassment. In clothes shops, on a beach, with friends, playing cricket, seeing people after a gap.

Depression. At lack of self-control, at evidence of middle-age, at knowledge of impaired health.

Gaining weight and being fat appeared to be my most intractable personal problem. I hated myself physically and despised my ineffectiveness. I didn't shape up. When I crossed the 180-pound line, self-respect or self-hatred would motivate me, and I'd go on another diet regime. Dieting was my dirty little secret. But my greed was a vice I couldn't keep to myself. It showed.

In 1978 the consumer magazine *Which?* surveyed 1001 slimmers, 788 women and 213 men. The main single reason given for failure as a dieter was 'lack of willpower and determination'. 'I know how to lose weight. I know I can lose weight. I lack the willpower to keep at it for what amounts to a lifetime, because whenever I give up on the programme I put it on again,' said one respondent. And another, 'I am very good at losing weight but once the loss slows down I give up and tend to put it all back on again.' As for me, two couplets by Theodore Roethke came to mind:

> Self-contemplation is a curse
> That makes an old confusion worse.
> He who himself begins to loathe
> Grows sick in flesh and spirit both.

But what to do? I ate, I wanted food, I grew fat. Food, hunger, appetite, my body, were my enemies.

Too much energy in, too little out

Diet books usually say that fat people either eat too much or take too little exercise. That seems common sense enough. So, I thought, maybe my vice was not greed, but sloth. Most diet books do not, however, forecast a slim future for the fat exerciser. 'It is extremely difficult to lose significant weight by exercise,' says Dr Tarnower. 'A half hour of energetic bicycling, for instance, uses up 200-280 calories, which you put right back on by eating an iced cupcake.' And Dr Stillman: 'even walking at moderate speed for a full hour uses only about 200 calories; no amount of exercising will reduce you if you over-eat.'

Professor Yudkin looks kindly upon exercise but says, nevertheless, that 'to dispose of a single cheese sandwich you would have to play squash for an hour. And to dispose of a good business lunch, you would have to play squash for eight hours.' At a press conference held by the Obesity Research Foundation in London in August 1982, Derek Miller of Queen Elizabeth College repeated the claim made in diet books that to get rid of the energy content of a hearty meal it would be necessary to walk up and down Ben Nevis.

The message was clear, for me. Fat people eat too much. Slim people do not hike up Britain's highest mountain after dinner, nor do they get on their bikes after eating a cupcake. The harm was in greed, not in sloth.

Diet books get their information from textbooks. A calorie as defined by a standard work of reference is:

A unit in which energy is measured. Technically, a calorie is the amount of heat necessary to raise the temperature of a gram of water one degree Centigrade. Food energy is measured in kilocalories.

(A kilocalorie is 1000 calories. But most people, nutritionists included, refer to a kilocalorie simply as a calorie.) Research on the energy value of food and of exercise started at the end of the nineteenth century. Nutrition textbooks now give calorie values of snack foods. So:

	measure	calories
Cupcake (chocolate, iced)	2¾ inches diameter	185
Sandwiches:		
Cheddar cheese	1 sandwich	280

It seems that Dr Tarnower favoured a large cupcake.

Other textbooks, on exercise physiology, give the calorie value of every kind of exercise for people of different weights (the more you weigh, the more energy you use up in any activity). Below are figures for a 'standard' eight stone eight woman and eleven stone man as listed in the text books:

	(minutes)	8 st 8 lb (cals)	11 st (cals)
Cycling (leisure, 9.4 mph)	30	168	213
Squash	60	714	916

It seems that Dr Tarnower was a fast cyclist. On the other hand, unless Professor Yudkin eats heroic sandwiches or plays a very leisurely game of squash, his figures are wildly wrong. However, his point can be made more modestly by proposing that a cheese sandwich (280 calories) takes an hour of walking off (270 calories for the eight stone eight woman, 342 calories for the eleven stone man). Dr John Garrow, in his book *Treat Obesity Seriously*, estimates that the fabled run of Pheidippides, the original marathon run to announce the victory of the Greeks over the Persians, cost him about 2500 calories. In the legend, Pheidippides died on arrival.

Calorie counting

Leaving exercise aside, I turned to the diet books that claimed that I could, by means of self-denial and their regime, lose ten pounds or more a week. In any case, I was a dieting expert. I believed the diet books; they worked. My problem was that after I stopped the diet I regained the weight I had lost. The fault, I was sure, was mine. I was a backslider. I was greedy.

What should I weigh? My ideal related to the tables of 'desirable body weight for men' published in books and magazines, and screwed on weighing-machines. These tables were devised by an American, Louis Dublin, for the Metropolitan Life Insurance Company. Dublin later decided to categorise people into arbitrary large-, medium- and small-frame sizes.

According to the tables my 'desirable' body weight,

at slightly over five foot eleven and a half inches and wearing indoor clothing, is:

Height	Small (pounds)	Frame Medium (pounds)	Large (pounds)
5 foot 11	144-154	150-165	159-179
6 foot	148-158	154-170	164-184

These 'desirable weights' varied from a little less than my heaviest weight ever to my lightest: nearly three stone. The range for a woman of average height is nearly two stone. I decided privately that 'large frame' was polite for 'fat' and that the tables were nonsense. Nor, in honest moments, did I go in for the idea that I had heavy bones. Nevertheless, the tables retained their fascination. I had a dream; I aspired to the bottom of the 'small-frame' scale. I had no idea of what the weight of my own body should be. I wanted to reduce myself to a statistic.

How much should I eat? Diet books rely on textbooks listing recommended energy intake, and these books in turn determine how much energy in the form of food should be produced and supplied to national and international populations. There is general agreement about human energy requirements. The US Government recommends that the energy intake of a 'standard' man of eleven stone and five foot ten inches tall who engages in 'light activity' should be:

Age	Daily calorie intake (range)
19-22	2500-3300
23-50	2300-3100
51-75	2000-2800
76 +	1650-2450

'Light activity' is defined as 'sleep or lie down for eight hours a day, sit for seven hours, stand for five, walk for two, and spend two hours a day in light physical activity', which summed me up well enough, in those days. 'For adults, it is believed that an 800 calorie range covers most individuals,' says one textbook. The energy requirements of the standard woman weighing eight stone eight pounds and five foot four tall are 1200 calories a day at the lowest end of the scale for a seventy-six-year-old, and 2500 calories a day at the top end of the scale for a nineteen- to twenty-two-year-old.

The bigger you are, the more energy you need. And the older you are, the less energy you need, because people tend to slow down as they get older.

This is why diet books tell you to cut down your energy intake from food to 1500 calories a day or less. Audrey Eyton, in *The F-Plan Diet*, says: 'Allow yourself 1500 calories daily if you are male, of at least medium height, and more than half a stone overweight . . . Allow yourself 1000 calories daily if you are female and less than one stone overweight.'

Dr Tarnower says, 'The Scarsdale Medical Diet averages 1000 calories or less a day.' Dr Stillman is very stern. 'You may falsify a calorie total on paper, but your body adds correctly and will turn into fat any extra calories that you omit by fake mathematics.' At one point he recommends a lettuce, lean meat and hard-boiled egg diet totaling 354 calories a day. Another Stillman diet, for the fainter-hearted, is the 'Six Meals-A-Day Nibbler Diet'. Of this he says, 'Whereas 900 to 1000 calories is the usual number allowed on a calorie-counting diet the nibbler diet allows you 1200 to 1800 calories a day.' This calorific cornucopia is against Dr Stillman's nature. 'For desirable quick weight loss,' he goes on, 'start with 900 to 1200 calories daily and then you may increase after you've learned control.'

Diet doctors tend to be stern. Dr Arnold Fox devised *The Beverly Hills Medical Diet* (BHMD; it has nothing to do with Judy Mazel's regime). 'Lose ten pounds in fourteen days! Enjoy potatoes, pasta and other forbidden foods', promises the front cover. But when Dr Fox comes to define what he calls 'freedom with responsibility' he says, 'You are permitted to mix different recipes and to redesign the menus according to your personal preferences – provided you don't exceed the 1200 calorie limit.' And he goes on: 'Consult the BHMD calorie chart to determine the calorie count of each recipe.'

'The fewer calories you consume, the more quickly you will lose weight – within limits,' writes Professor

Yudkin, and 'A daily 1000 calories is normally recommended as the safe low-calorie limit.' Whether diet books favour fibre (Eyton), protein (Stillman, Tarnower), carbohydrate (Fox) or oppose carbohydrate (Yudkin) the story is the same: lose weight by cutting calories, usually to 1000 – 1500 a day.

Dieters feel that their fat is their fault and that they are fat because they eat too much. Dieting is fuelled by guilt and self-disgust. Many dieters feel that the most conspicuous and inescapable evidence of their general failure to manage themselves and their world is their fat. Fat people believe that they are unfit and unhealthy. Hatred of being fat, and fear of becoming fat, are demoralising and disturbing to the point, for many dieters, of affecting their sanity. I know: I was there. I was alienated from my body; it was out of my control. Cyril Connolly wrote, 'Imprisoned in every fat man, a thin one is wildly signalling to be let out.' The thin being has been taken over; surrounded in the most literal way, by the alien, fat being.

Clearly, from what I had read, exercise could do little for me. The British Code of Advertising Practice on slimming aids confirms this view:

A diet is the only practicable self-treatment for achieving a reduction in excess fat . . . Claims, whether direct or indirect, that weight loss can be achieved by any other means are not acceptable.

But what to do? I dieted, I lost weight, I regained the weight, I grew fat. I was my own enemy.

Could it be greed?

Something that vaguely puzzled me at the time was that I didn't think I was eating all that much. 'Self-deceit!' say the diet doctors. An acquaintance of mine, a doctor who is a nutritionist with a busy private practice of fat patients who want to be thin, regards them as naughty children who need discipline: firm instructions, an ordered regime. Otherwise, he tells me, they'll always cheat. The usual fable of the health farm is of the delinquent fatties who lure their fellows in obesity over the perimeter at dead of night for a gastronomic orgy at the local five-star hotel.

11

Did I raid the refrigerator at night more often than other people? Were my portions larger, my meals bigger? Was I addicted to snacks? Diet books even include stories of people who go on sleep-walking binges. Could that be me? I watched friends and colleagues as we ate. They tucked in; they were not fat. I ate, feelings of self-disgust alternating with feelings of 'to hell with it'; I was fat. Was I really eating more than they were? Did they raid the refrigerator? Did they buy chocolate bars on the way home? These are questions you don't ask. But why was I never rewarded by my bouts of dieting? The great card-sharp in the sky seemed to have stacked the deck against me.

Some people do, indeed, eat compulsively, and thereby become obese. I had the impression that the average fat person was a big eater – why else should people get fat? – and that gargantuan appetite led to obesity. For a man, the images are of two kings, Henry VIII and Edward VII: the one throwing gnawed haunches of venison over his shoulder; the other gobbling breakfasts of partridge pie, cold mutton, truffles, a dozen plover's eggs and kedgeree, washed down with a pint of claret.

While not having such a regal appetite, I assumed that my problem was greed. But my assumption was contradicted by the measurement of the energy equivalent of fat on which all diet books base their calculations. Diet books start from the position that the energy equivalent of a pound of fat is 3500 calories (or, to use the exact term, 'kcal'). Thus, Audrey Eyton, in *The F-Plan Diet*, instancing a woman whose normal energy requirement is 2000 calories a day:

> If we were to put you on a slimming diet providing you with 1500 calories a day, you would be 500 calories short of your requirement and these would have to be taken from your body fat. It has been scientifically estimated that a pound of your own body fat provides approximately 3500 calories. So during a week you would be likely to shed one pound of surplus fat.

And, by the same calculation, anyone who not only abandons the F-Plan but also consumes 500 calories too many will gain one pound of surplus fat every week.

John Durnin, Professor of Physiology at the University of Glasgow, has told me that this calculation is inaccurate. It is based on laboratory experiments made 100 years ago that do not take account of the biochemistry within the human body. He says that

> losing one pound of fat would result in a net energy deficit nearer 3000 kcal. More important, because the mechanical and biochemical efficiency of depositing adipose [fatty] tissue is relatively inefficient, you need about 4500 kcal to lay down one pound of fat in the body.

A tangerine too many?

Allowing for Professor Durnin's correction, a reminder that human chemistry is more subtle than the chemistry conducted in laboratories on inert material, then many of us would indeed be gross. An extra 4500 calories a week is just under 650 calories a day. According to Dr Fox's BHMD Diet, 650 calories may be composed of:

Hamburger, broiled, regular, 3oz	245
Potato crisps, 2 in diameter, 10 crisps	115
Beer, 12 fl oz (2)	300

Or, from a standard textbook:

Chocolate, plain (3.5 oz)	525
Peanuts, salted (25 gm)	150

Or, from Audrey Eyton's *F-Plan Calorie and Fibre Chart*:

Cake, fruit, plain, average slice (2)	400
Biscuit, digestive wheatmeal (4)	280

So, according to these figures, and on the diet books' arithmetic, a couple of snacks a day over the odds in a cafe, bar or at home will result in the consumption of food with an energy content of 650 calories or more.

In this case, if the diet books are to be believed, anyone who eats this quantity of food surplus to their daily requirements will gain one pound of fat a week, which is

13

to say over fifty pounds a year, or over 500 every ten years.

I seemed to gain about twelve pounds a year. It was difficult to be precise, since, when not on a diet, I was usually making up weight lost from the previous diet.

The weekly equivalent of twelve pounds a year is near enough four ounces. Given that these four ounces are fat, the caloric equivalent – allowing for Professor Durnin's correction of the textbook figures – is 1125 a week, or 160 a day, extra to my requirement.

So, if my problem was, indeed, that I was eating 160 calories a day too many, the answer should be simple. According to the diet books, I should be able to maintain a steady weight by every day saying 'no' to any of the following, give or take the odd calorie:

Sweet biscuits, 1 oz (2)	160-170	(*Which?*)
Yoghurt, low-fat, hazel-nut, 5.3 oz	160	(Eyton)
Martini	150	(Stillman)
Gingerbread, 2 × 2 × 2 in (1)	180	(Tarnower)
Wine, dessert (4 oz glass)	160	(Fox)

It is difficult to wrap the brain around the notion that one glass of wine (or one pint of beer) over the odds is evidence of greed. Furthermore, a weight gain of twelve pounds a year is 120 pounds a decade, an increase that would take me from an initial post-diet weight of eleven stone seven pounds, say, to twenty stone. That, of course, was what I feared, the fate to which I believed I was doomed, unless I dieted. British weighing-machines often stop at eighteen stone. The thought of going off the scale was a waking nightmare.

The fact is, though, that people who gain fat do not do so at anything like the rate of 120 pounds a decade. A more typical rate of increase, for the man or woman who in time becomes over-fat, and one of the sixty-five per cent of British women or thirty per cent of British men who (according to the Royal College of Physicians in 1983) try to lose weight each year, would not be one hundred and twenty pounds a decade but perhaps thirty pounds. This would change the slim young woman aged twenty weighing eight stone, into a woman aged twenty-five weighing just over nine stone, and into one of thirty weighing over ten stone who will be worrying about her weight. Likewise, a man who between the ages of twenty and thirty increased from eleven stone to over thirteen stone, would metamorphose from being slim to being decidedly overweight and liable to worry about becoming obese in the next decade. (These figures assume sedentary women and men of average height; taller people might gain rather more weight proportionally from a heavier initial weight.)

The energy equivalent of a gain of thirty pounds of fat in a decade is forty calories of energy from food a day. Forty calories a day? The diet books count them:

Potato crisps, 2 in diameter, (4)	46	(Fox)
Tangerine, raw, 2 ½ in diameter	40	(Tarnower)
Butter, 1 pat	50	(Stillman)
Pickle, sweet, 1 oz (1 rounded tbsp)	40	(Eyton)
Tomatoes, fried, 2 oz	40-50	(*Which?*)

Most diet books recommend calorie control. Theirs is a world where the dieter is invited to measure potato crisps with a ruler and to believe that eating four more than the body's requirements will lead to a weight gain of thirty pounds in a decade (to be exact, close to thirty-five pounds according to Dr Fox's calculations, assuming that the crisps are round and not elliptical). And eating three less than requirement – a difference of seven crisps – will lead to a weight loss of thirty pounds in a decade.

No diet book has ever made such a claim, because it is absurd. But there it is: the arithmetic, supposedly based on science, proposes that one tangerine too many, every day, is the path to obesity. Can such a notion possibly be true?

Three crisps too few?

Consider the arithmetic for the person who eats three crisps too few each day. (This amounts to a two-ounce packet of crisps too few once a week.) The consequent and apparently inexorable weight loss would mean that the slim young woman of nine stone aged twenty would weigh two stone eight pounds aged fifty. If she underdid it not by three but by four crisps a day, by the age of fifty she would have disappeared altogether.

Consider a different case: the person who does eat or

15

drink quite a lot too much. Take, say, the man who puts away three pints of beer and a couple of packets of peanuts a day, on top of eating and drinking enough for his body's needs. (If that is greed, there is a lot of it about.) This extra intake, with a pint of bitter at 175 calories and peanuts at 300 calories a fifty-gram packet, is 1125 calories a day. At that rate, the '4500 calories equals one pound of fat' equation implies that this moderate drinker would gain about eight pounds a month, or just under 100 pounds every year.

Professor Durnin cites the case of William Campbell, the Scot who died aged twenty-two in 1878 having established the United Kingdom record for obesity, at 341 kg. 'We can estimate,' says Durnin:

> that in his 22 years he acquired fat representing an excess over intake of about 1 ¾ million kcal. If we now calculate what average daily excess would be required to achieve his record-breaking weight in 22 years, the answer comes to 218 kcal a day.

And, Durnin goes on to point out, well aware that his fellow-Scots are known to drink a pint or two a day and even eat the odd peanut: 'Differences of this magnitude, of 200 kcal, are frequently found between measurements of the average daily intake and the energy expenditure of the individual.' In which case, what can overweight have to do with greed?

In my dieting days, I never did the sums necessary to show that the reasoning of the diet books advocating calorie control was preposterous. Although calorie counting did strike me as obsessive to the point of being deranged, I took the books on trust. After all, every diet I went on worked. They succeeded. I failed.

I was also concerned about my health. The diet books have ways of keeping the dieter obedient. Dr Stillman has a chapter entitled 'Facts to Help "Scare" the Fat off You'. He quotes Brillat-Savarin. 'Well, go ahead and eat and grow fat,' the French gourmet said. 'Become ugly, heavy, have asthmatic attacks and die choked by your own fat.' Or, according to Stillman, Tarnower, and indeed *Which? Way to Slim*, suffer or die from diabetes, gall-stones, arthritis, strokes, heart disease. 'If you're ten per cent overweight,' says Stillman 'you'll lose seven years of living. In effect you will have committed suicide at sixty-three.' I did not want to suffer or die prematurely. What was the matter with me? Could I be saved?

Fat people eat less

John Garrow is often cited as the leading authority on obesity in England. He wrote in 1974 that there is 'no evidence of any relationship between energy intake and body weight in man'. In 1977 at a congress on obesity he said that no evidence had been found 'that obese people ate more than thin ones. The cause of obesity is astonishingly difficult to pin down.' I asked Dr Garrow if any evidence had emerged since 1977 to show that fat people ate more than thin people. He said no.

In 1974 Professor Durnin, in a study made in Glasgow, found that fat girls did not eat more than thin girls: they ate less than thin girls. Durnin also made two studies of fourteen-year-old boys and girls, in 1964 and 1971. Calorie intake had fallen by 180 to 250 calories a day during the seven years. In 1971 the boys who were eating less were fatter than the 1964 boys. (Girls stayed much the same.) In 1982 Durnin published similar findings for babies. Nutritionist Alison Paul and others undertook a variation of this study in 1982 and discovered that today's teenagers eat fewer calories than their parents and, indeed, eat 300 to 500 calories a day less than is recommended by the World Health Organisation. But nevertheless they tend to be overweight.

In 1979 Professor Harry Keen reported on a study of links between what and how much people eat, and diabetes. As part of his study he measured the amount of food people ate, and their degree of fatness, in three population samples: 961 employees of Beechams Foods; 1005 employees of the Greater London Council; and 1488 middle-aged male civil servants. What he found, to his surprise, was 'highly significant inverse correlations between food energy intake and adiposity [degree of fatness], a relation found in both sexes and in all three population samples.'

17

That is to say, the fatter people were eating less than the thinner people. This applied to both men and women and to all the groups studied. Keen eliminated people who were slimming from his analysis; this did not affect his results. He considered the possibility that the fatter people were underestimating how much they were eating; but such self-deception is only likely among people worried about being fat, and Keen's study was of people who did not see themselves as having a weight problem. Also, Keen's discovery that thinner people ate more and that fatter people ate less applied right across the range of thinness and fatness, not just to those people who were most overweight. As was to be expected, Keen found that people got fatter as they got older; but the rule that fatter people ate less and thinner people ate more applied to all ages.

The Royal College of Physicians, commenting in their 1983 report on obesity on surveys of British men and women done in the last fifty years, states: 'There now seems little doubt that there is a general trend for both men and women to become heavier and presumably fatter, this change being particularly evident in young adults.'

As officially measured in 1981, the proportion of British people carrying excess weight is about a quarter of men and women in their twenties and just under a half of men and women over the age of forty. The figures are

Age	Men	Women
	(Percentage with excess weight)	
16 – 19	15	15
20 – 24	22	23
25 – 29	29	20
30 – 39	40	25
40 – 49	52	38
50 – 59	49	47
60 – 65	54	50
Total	39	32

The estimated amount of body fat has also risen steadily in the last twenty years.

But the *National Food Survey*, an official publication, shows that the amount of energy consumed from food has steadily dropped in the last twenty years. In 1960 the British people were consuming 2628 calories a day from food. In 1981 the figure had dropped to 2210: a fall of nineteen per cent. The figures for recent years are

1960	1965	1970	1975	1979	1980	1981
2628	2590	2560	2290	2250	2230	2210

These figures exaggerate the drop in energy intake from food because they do not reflect the fact that there are now more old people, who tend to eat less, than there were in 1960. They also do not take into account food eaten outside the home; and consumption of snack food has risen in the 1970s. The Ministry of Agriculture publishes statistics of food imported and produced in Britain before it is processed. These figures do not allow for the waste of food in manufacture and thereafter, but they do include food eaten outside the home. They show that consumption of sugar reached a peak in 1977 and that alcohol consumption is continuing to rise; and that overall there was a drop of 222 calories a day energy from food consumed between 1960 and 1981.

Whatever the exact figure may be, it is safe to say that we are getting fatter while eating less. Professor Peter Wood of Stanford University confirms that the same is true in the USA and adds, referring to findings from the USA, Britain and other Western countries, 'These facts relate to an interesting finding from several large population studies; generally speaking fatter people eat less than thinner people.'

But if over-eating is not the cause of obesity, so that the very word 'obese' (derived from *ob* – 'over' and *edere* – 'to eat') is based on a misconception, what makes people fat? If not gluttony, then what? The answer seemed to lie in a word not much mentioned in the diet books but which has crept into many women's magazine features lately: 'metabolism'. The Obesity Research Foundation says:

The ability of some people to eat what they like and not gain weight is the constant envy of the obese. It would seem that the lean and the obese are metabolically different, and the explanation of the difference is an urgent challenge to science.

My granny used to say that fat people had something wrong with their glands; I thought this was a homely way of saying, as is often said now, that fat people have 'a low metabolism' or, more correctly, 'a low metabolic rate'. Was this my doom? Had the great double-dealer in the sky given me an unwinnable hand? Should fat people not be scorned as greedy, but pitied as helpless?

Eating like a bird and like a horse

The notion that fat people are lumbered with a low metabolism has been popularised by Dr Robert C Atkins, whose *Diet Revolution*, *Super-Energy Diet* and *Nutrition Breakthrough* have sold a total of twelve million books, world-wide. Dr Atkins is as enthusiastic about his books as Dr Stillman and Dr Tarnower were about theirs. He maintains that:

> Failure to lose weight on a diet low in both calories and carbohydrates is strong evidence of a metabolic imbalance . . . variations in metabolic responses are important factors in obesity, and any physician should know that he will be seeing many cases of impaired response.

Metabolism can be defined as 'the sum total of all the chemical reactions that go on in living cells'. Metabolic rate is the speed at which the body uses energy, which it needs for the constant process of replacing and renewing cells in all its parts while asleep and at rest; for the digestion of food; and for activity. Most people use most energy not for activity but for the workings of their vital organs – the brain, heart, liver and kidneys especially. Put simply, metabolic rate is the speed at which our bodies work.

It is commonplace, nowadays, for people to describe themselves as having either (luckily) a 'high metabolism' or (unluckily) a 'low metabolism'. The assumption is that we are stuck with the metabolic rate with which we are born. The fault is not in ourselves – in our sloth, or greed, or both – but in our genes. (Indeed, people more sophisticated than my gran use 'genes' rather than 'glands' as an excuse for obesity.)

20

Interestingly, this determinist proposition is similar to the now discredited theory that we are stuck with the intelligence (IQ) with which we are born. It takes away a sense of personal responsibility for our physical shape and blames the Almighty, or heredity. In my case, my father is over-fat, whereas his father was lean; so I half-believed that when the chromosomal dice were cast I got the low metabolic numbers. I was a slow burner; I was one of those who gained weight as soon as I 'looked at a bun', because I had a low metabolism. My friends and colleagues who ate heartily but evidently gained no weight had a high metabolism.

One analogy for metabolism is engine capacity. Thus, a middle-aged woman may have a Mini-Minor capacity and so eat 'like a bird' and yet be plump; whereas a young man with a Range-Rover capacity can 'eat like a horse' and yet stay lean. And, just as Mini-Minors do not turn into Range-Rovers, nor birds into horses, the inference is that metabolic rate is inborn. Analogies always carry inferences.

Another analogy often used for human metabolism is the central heating system. Hence the concept of the 'appestat'. Yudkin says: 'You could more or less describe the appestat as the part of the brain that controls how much we eat in the same way that a thermostat controls temperature.' But 'if you are overweight, you don't stop wanting to eat when you've had enough. So obviously something has gone wrong with your appestat.' The thermostat that controls the temperature of my bath-water is set at 175°F, just as the thermostatic mechanism that controls the temperature of my body is set at 98.4°F.

If I now go to my water-heater and turn the thermostat up to 185°F, I shall quite soon become too hot, because the heater is also part of my central heating system. If the heater's thermostat jammed at 185°F, it would be too high and would have gone wrong. With this analogy in mind, a number of scientists, aware that fat people do not characteristically eat more than thin people, have proposed the 'set-point' theory. This supposes that people who tend to obesity suffer from a condition in which the mechanism that regulates their body weight is set too high. As a result they tend to gain weight.

A champion of 'set-point' theory is Professor Richard Keesey of the University of Wisconsin. Keesey works with rats. He says:

> Laboratory animals, like human beings, appear to regulate body weight around a stable level or set-point. If their weight is reduced by restricting their calorie intake, rats rapidly restore body weight to the level of nonrestricted controls when allowed to feed freely . . . Thus, as in man, the stability and vigorous defence of its body weight by the rat suggest the presence of a set-point regulator.

That is to say, I was born to be fat. The implication of this ingenious theory is that my weight, when I was dieting, was never meant to fluctuate; that it went down – and then up – because I dieted; and that if I left well alone and ate what I wanted, my weight would stop at some point, and stay steady at that 'set' point.

Born to be fat?

In *The Dieter's Dilemma* Dr William Bennett and Joel Gurin have popularised set-point theory. They say:

> Some individuals come with a high setting, others with a low one. Some are therefore naturally fat and others thin. Going on a diet is an attempt to overpower the body's set-point; it is not a fair contest. The set-point is a tireless opponent.

'Your setting,' they go on, 'is the weight you normally maintain, give or take a few points, when you are not thinking about it.'

'The set-point theory is, admittedly, somewhat fatalistic,' say Bennett and Gurin. But it does have charm. It suggests that the dieter's problem is not becoming fat but refusing to accept that she or he is designed by nature to be fat. Love it! 'The obsessive drive to be thin serves no real purpose, except to funnel large amounts of money into the diet industry,' they say. And: 'The prejudice against fatness is cruel, destructive, and unfair.' They find support from the 'Fat is Beautiful' movement in the USA and also from Susie Orbach, whose book *Fat is a Feminist*

Issue quite rightly sees tyranny in the pressure put on women to become super slim.

Was there, then, truth in what my granny told me? Was I born to be fat?

Set-point theory cannot explain why the average body fat content of the British adult population has increased by ten per cent in the last forty years. (Statistics from the USA are similar.) Set-point theory, the darling of many writers in America, falls to the ground. It has to be far-fetched. In any case, is it true that 'most of us remain on essentially the same body weight', as set-point theory proposes?

No, it isn't. Set-point theory was discredited before many people had heard of it, let alone believed it. In 1974 a survey of long-stay prisoners in Wormwood Scrubs, whose body weight was measured annually in the eight years between 1965 and 1972, was published in *Obesity and Energy Balance in Man*, a book by Dr John Garrow, who explained:

> It may be that long-stay prisoners are not typical of the general population, but on general grounds one might expect that their weight would be more stable than that of the population at liberty; their way of life is more like that of laboratory animals which show great stability of body weight.

And the results of the routine weighing of these prisoners? 'On average their weight varied over a range of seven and a half kg [sixteen and a half pounds] during a period of seven years.'

Garrow supported his findings by quoting studies of more than 1000 people in Wales over four years, which showed weight deviations of over twenty pounds; and of the community of Framingham in the USA in which 'on average, both men and women fluctuated by ten kg [twenty-two pounds] over eighteen years.'

So much for set-point theory. Man is not a rat. In 1976, my last year of dieting, I was not aware of set-point theory, but I was no closer than its champions have ever been to finding out why I got fat. If the reason wasn't sloth, and wasn't greed, and wasn't genes, what could it be?

In his *Super-Energy Diet* Dr Atkins calls a chapter 'If You Are Not Getting Results'. Addressed to hopeless cases, it includes a tip which sounds the most loony but harmless remedy for the overweight ever proposed. 'A surefire trick if you can afford it,' he says, is to 'go to Europe'. How could this help me? I live in Europe. But Dr Atkins perseveres:

> For some strange reason, as yet unexplained, a trip to Europe always seems to help with weight reduction. It may be something in the soil . . . The best results seem to be achieved in Mediterranean countries: Spain, Greece, Italy, or the south of France.

In summer 1979 I had not read Dr Atkins, and I had abandoned dieting, having decided that I'd rather get fat than go mad. I went on holiday to Greece for a month to Antiparos, a tiny island in the Cyclades. When I left England, I weighed a flabby twelve stone twelve. When I returned I was down eight pounds at twelve stone four. I later lost a bit more weight, while eating and drinking whatever I want. For the first time in my life my weight has been stable.

What had happened in Greece? Its clean air had given me a good appetite, and this book does not propose that eating makes you thin.

Exercise: the key?

Nor was the reason that I was taking more exercise than usual. The reverse was true – for the previous autumn I had started to jog. I had been in Hyde Park, watching the first *Sunday Times* National Fun Run. The exaltation of the runners, some almost twice my age, was an inspiration – not to start running to lose weight, but to join in running, to participate. Watching the runners, and reflecting on an imminent fortieth birthday, I came to three conclusions: I was a spectator of, not a participant in, my own life; there are no easy ways out, and nothing worthwhile is easy; and if I didn't start then, I never would.

So I started to jog. By the next summer I was doing gentle four and a half mile runs and sometimes covered twenty miles in a week. Then came the Greek holiday, during, which I enjoyed walking, and some swimming, and a sense of well-being earned by my new fitness that I'd never experienced before as an adult. But I took no more, and probably less, exercise on that holiday than in the previous months. Afterwards I regarded the weight loss as an enigma.

Since then, running has become part of my life. I still weigh twelve stone, but I have changed shape. And talking with many people about the effect of exercise on weight and fat I have found plenty who, like me, started running when ten to thirty pounds overfat, lost weight, lost fat, and now eat and drink what they like. It was when I realised that I would never again have to diet that I started the research for this book.

CHAPTER TWO

Dieting Makes You Fat

The Holy Grail of Western medicine is a safe and
comfortable way to lose excessive body fat. This fruitless
search has been the basis of an almost endless array of
'reducing diets' that have tantalised the fat folks and
enriched the publishers and the medical businessmen. The
reducing diets have been disappointing – some would say,
a medical disaster.
GEORGE MANN
New England Journal of Medicine

It was not through statements that we learned how to
breathe, swallow, see, circulate the blood, digest food, or
resist diseases. Yet these things are performed by the most
complex and marvellous processes which no amount of
booklearning and technical skill can reproduce. But we
have been taught to neglect, despise and violate our bodies,
and to put all our faith in our brains. As a consequence, we
are at war within ourselves – the brain desiring things
which the body does not want, and the body desiring
things which the brain does not allow; the brain giving
directions which the body will not follow, and the body
giving impulses which the brain cannot understand.
ALAN WATTS
The Wisdom of Insecurity

The big slow down

A successful diet book is liable to sell millions of copies
world-wide. People who want to lose weight do not try to
do so for fun. For many people, their desire to lose weight
matters as much as anything else in their lives.

Dieters are entitled to expect that any writer of a diet

book will have at least an elementary knowledge of the effects of dieting on the human body. As a rule, diet books are based on two assumptions about dieting. First, that diets do not affect the speed at which the body works – the metabolic rate. Second, that weight lost on a diet is all or almost all fat. 'When you are slimming you are really eating your own body – eating away the part of it you don't want, that surplus fat!' says Audrey Eyton.

It is a pity to single out Mrs Eyton, because her F-Plan recommends eating foods rich in fibre, which often are nourishing, whereas the foods recommended by other diet books are often disgusting, debilitating or even dangerous. But she is typical of writers of diet books when she says, having made the 'one pound of body fat equals 3500 calories' calculation, that:

> Expected rate of fat loss has always been estimated simply by counting the calories consumed in the form of food, any food, and subtracting them from the number the body requires for energy . . . With a daily deficit of 1000 calories you could expect to shed around two pounds a week.

But is it true that diets do not affect the speed at which the body works? No, it is not. Diets slow down the metabolic rate. And is it true that weight lost on diets is fat or almost all fat? No, it is not. Much of the weight lost on a diet is not fat; and any initial fast weight loss is not because of removal of fat.

These facts have been known for many years. Research into the effect of diets on the body started at the beginning of this century and has been repeated again and again. The silence of diet books on the effects of dieting on the body is so total, and the profits to be made from them are so large, that it is impossible to believe that all diet books are written in good faith. They lead readers to believe that when diets fail it is the dieter who is to blame. Of course they do; the writer of a diet book doesn't want the reader to doubt the book, and self-doubt helps diet book sales. In fact, diets fail because of what they do to the body of the dieter.

What happens to the body of a dieter depends to a considerable extent on the nature, severity and length of the diet, and also on the body composition, eating habits and way of life of the dieter.

First, any diet book that claims or suggests that an initial weight loss of ten to fifteen pounds a week is of fat is misleading the reader, as a simple calculation will show. The energy required to burn off a pound of body fat is 3000 calories (Professor Durnin's correct figure). It follows that the energy required to burn off ten to fifteen pounds of fat a week is 30,000 to 45,000 calories, or 4286 to 6429 calories a day. But diet regimes recommend cutting down by 500 to 1500 calories a day. There is thus no way that the initial fast weight loss, which dieters are led to believe is proof of success, can be of body fat. Simple mathematics prove the point.

(Some of the more reckless writers of diet books, usually those first published in the USA, suggest that the foods recommended on their regimes have a special fat-burning property in addition to their low-calorie value. These claims are nonsense; they have the same sort of relationship to nutrition as astrology does to astronomy.)

Rapid weight loss is of glycogen

The body's first reaction to a diet regime is to draw on the energy that is immediately available in any emergency. This is not fat; the body has no means to make immediate use of its fat. The body's immediately available form of energy is a substance that you do not read about in diet books: glycogen. Glycogen is a form of glucose (a carbohydrate) stored in solution with water in the muscles and in the body's most metabolically active vital organ, the liver.

How much glycogen does the body contain? It is difficult to be exactly sure. Unlike other constituents of the body (bone, or fat, for example) it cannot be dissected, because it disappears after death; and this is a reason why its function has tended to be overlooked until recently. The Scandinavian physiologists Professor Per-Olof Åstrand and Professor Bengt Saltin have made a special study of glycogen. I asked them, and also Dr John Garrow, to make an estimate of the body's glycogen content. These three authorities were in broad agreement. First, the body stores glycogen in solution, in the proportion 1:2.7 glycogen to water; second, the amount of 'solid' glycogen the body contains is in the region of two pounds. It follows from this that the weight of glycogen in solution contained in the body, is approximately seven and a half pounds.

Glycogen burns very much faster than fat. The energy value of carbohydrate is approximately four-ninths that of fat. Given that the energy required to burn off a pound of body fat is 3000 calories, the figure for 'solid' glycogen is 1333 calories, and for glycogen in solution with water, around 400 calories, a pound. (Only a little energy is required to release water from the body's cells.)

So, initial rapid weight loss on a diet is no mystery. The loss is principally of glycogen bound up with water, and also of additional water. Simple mathematics prove the point. This otherwise inexplicable rapid weight loss is a familiar phenomenon in sport. A footballer playing hard in the sun, or a marathon runner, can lose up to ten pounds, or even more, in two or three hours. I myself have lost eight pounds running a half-marathon on a humid day.

A special diet used by marathon runners (the so-called 'carbohydrate-bleeding' regime) consists of food specially designed to drain the glycogen stores, and loses about six pounds in three days. It is not a calorie-controlled diet: you can eat as much as you like of very high-protein foods such as meat, fish, eggs and cheese. (The runners then follow the 'bleeding' regime with 'carbohydrate-loading' for the three days before a marathon, and saturate their bodies with energy-giving starch.)

The effect is the same as the diet regimes of Dr Stillman and Dr Tarnower, which recommend high protein and low carbohydrate; and of Dr Atkins, which recommends high fat and low carbohydrate. It is these diets which drain the body's own carbohydrate store – glycogen – fastest. The body must have carbohydrate: the brain, for example, uses glucose released into the blood almost exclusively as a fuel and has practically no glucose store of its own.

Low-carbohydrate diets drain the body's glycogen

stores in the first few days without touching the body's fat stores at all. Any diet regime that cuts calories by means of cutting sugars and starches – the carbohydrates – will have this effect. The Royal College of Physicians recognised the phenomenon in their 1983 report on obesity, stating of diet regimes that:

> The patient needs to know that short-term rapid weight losses with rigorous diets depend on losses of body water (with glycogen and protein) rather than on losses of body fat.

Low glycogen levels trigger the mechanism in the body that signals hunger. Food such as bread, spaghetti, cereals, beans and potatoes are satisfying not just because of their energy content but because they are rich in starch, a nutritious carbohydrate, that feeds the glycogen stores, raises the blood glucose level, and gives a sense of fullness and well-being.

By contrast, a runner on the 'carbohydrate-bleeding' regime eats lots of protein and, with a full stomach, loses weight and becomes ravenously, obsessively hungry, thinking of little else but food. This hunger has nothing to do with an empty stomach or a low energy intake, nor is it caused by loss of fat. The cause, and the cause of the weight loss, is exhaustion of the glycogen store, together with water. Exactly the same happens to dieters who cut down or cut out carbohydrates – starches and sugars. The surest way to get someone obsessed with food is to put them on a diet regime.

Glycogen loss leads to low blood-sugar levels. The result is a sense of weakness, depression, irritation, tiredness, and sometimes faintness and dizziness. Dieters will recognise the pattern.

At the same time as losing glycogen bound up with water, dieters also lose water from elsewhere in the body. It is possible to lose seven pounds of water sweating it out all night in a Turkish bath; I once won a lose-weight contest that way. Boxers and jockeys dehydrate themselves so as to weigh in under a required weight. The human body contains fifty to sixty-five per cent water. Women's bodies contain less water than men's, because body fat contains only a small amount of water, and the average woman has more fat than the average man. For the same reason, a fat person's body contains less water than that of a lean person of the same weight. Almost half our body weight is water contained within the body's cells. Water is essential for the body's metabolic processes. The body adapts to a diet by reducing the water content inside and outside the body's cells.

Fat people stay fat

In our minds we know the difference between going on a diet and being subjected to famine or starvation. But our bodies do not know the difference. When we go on a diet regime we activate the mechanisms in the body that protect us and preserve us in times of famine. And what does the body need to keep it going between times of famine? Fat. The more often people diet, the more their bodies will protect the stores of fat.

The human body can adapt to circumstances. It can get used to very hot or very cold weather, or to high altitude. The body constantly adjusts to accommodate a person's way of life, preserving what that person needs, if necessary at the expense of what is not needed, or at least not used.

Once a dieter's body has adapted to the diet by releasing glycogen and shedding water, it will then tend to lose the tissue it needs least.

The protein loss referred to by the Royal College of Physicians means loss of lean tissue, including muscle. Diet regimes also have the effect of wasting lean body tissue. If the diet is severe or takes the form of a fast, much or even most tissue lost will be lean body tissue, including muscle.

The body of a sedentary dieter will tend to lose lean tissue, muscle in particular, simply because a sedentary person does not need much muscle. The longer the dieter has been sedentary, the stronger the tendency for lean tissue to be lost. And the body of a fat dieter will seek to preserve fat, simply because it is accustomed to fat.

By contrast, the body of an active and relatively lean person, even if it has a large bulk of muscle, will tend to lose body fat, simply because the body has been trained to need muscle; it is being used all the time.

There comes a point, even in an almost inert person, at which the body will protect its lean tissue. But this switch takes some time. Doctors can devise diets for anyone which, with persistence, will lose far more fat than lean tissue. But the body's processes include what can be termed 'tissue memory'. After a time, interpreted as a crisis, the body will tend to rebuild itself in the form appropriate to the uses to which it is put.

Lean, active people who go on a diet – boxers and jockeys for example – lose weight efficiently, lose fat if they have any to lose, eat a lot after dieting to keep their bright fires burning, and tend to gain muscle, the body having adapted to their way of life. (Heavyweight boxers who go to fat do so because in training they may be so active that they can eat up to 7000 calories a day. Out of training they often continue to eat a great deal of food without being sufficiently active to consume the energy from it.)

Most dieters are not boxers or jockeys but are fat, inactive people. When fat inactive people diet, their bodies adapt to the diet not according to what they have in mind but according to their way of life. They tend to lose relatively more lean tissue, which is not needed on their life's voyage.

To sum up: dieting, of the type recommended in diet books, results in loss of glycogen, water and lean tissue from the body. And loss of glycogen causes the hunger, fatigue and depression that dieters experience.

Adapting to a diet

Dieting also slows the body down. First of all, a dieter is likely to become less active without necessarily even noticing. You may sleep a little longer, walk up stairs less often, not feel like tackling an energetic task, find that the television programmes have suddenly become very good, or just spend more time sitting and musing. In these situations the dieter is often not aware that a pattern of inactivity is forming, the means whereby the body seeks to make do with less food.

32

Equally, a dieter may also be conscious of becoming less active – 'I'm taking it easy, I'm on a diet'. The result may be a pleasant sense of restfulness or an unpleasant sense of lassitude. For the body, the results are the same.

Dieters do not normally take to their beds. During any but the most rigorous diet, activity is not usually dramatically reduced. But a man might use 150 to 450 calories a day less on activity, depending on whether he was sedentary or fairly active; a woman maybe 100 to 300 less.

Also, the less food you eat, the less energy you need to digest it. A diet that cuts 500 calories a day needs about fifty calories a day less energy for digestion. It follows, therefore, that if fairly active people cut 500 calories a day, their bodies need not lose significant amounts of fat, or of any other body tissue. The body of a fairly active person can adapt to a moderate diet by becoming the body of a sedentary person.

In practice people on a mild diet, if they keep to it, will lose some weight and also some fat. But they cannot lose a pound of fat a week by cutting 500 calories of food a day, or anything like that amount, unless they consciously compensate for the body's adaptation to the diet by becoming more active.

The reason why diet books specify an energy intake of 1000 calories a day from food for women and 1500 calories a day for men (or levels of this order) is because the body needs more energy than this for its basic, vital functions.

At rest, it is the vital organs that have most work to do. The brain accounts for about twenty per cent of the body's energy used at rest. The liver is even more active, accounting for about twenty-seven per cent of the body's activity at rest. The contribution of various parts of the resting body to energy turnover are estimated to be as follows:

Liver (and associated areas)	27 per cent
Brain	20
Heart	7
Kidneys	10
Skeletal muscle	18
Remainder	18

33

At rest, then, about sixty-five per cent of the energy the body needs is used by vital organs whose weight totals about five per cent of the body's weight. Of the remaining thirty-five per cent, some is used by body fat, which is not inert but, like the rest of the body, requires nourishment and constantly renews itself. Most of the remaining energy is used by muscle, which is more active than body fat. How much more active depends on the condition of the muscle. The little-used muscles of a sedentary person are relatively inactive at rest. Muscle regularly used, say by someone who exercises vigorously three or four times a week, is relatively active at all times, not just during exercise. This is because the stress of exercise breaks down muscle tissue, and the muscle then actively regenerates. During exercise, the energy used by muscle increases dramatically, by twenty, fifty or even a hundred times more than the amount used at rest, depending on the condition of the muscles and the intensity of the exercise.

The regularly used muscles of an active person are, with training, able to use more and more energy, and to burn more and more fat.

A sedentary person's body uses most of its energy from food for the vital autonomous functions (which happen unconsciously). In addition, the average healthy able-bodied sedentary person in the West will need maybe a quarter as much again energy, for the processes of conscious living: sitting down, talking, writing; and somewhat more energetic activities, such as standing, walking around the house and the office; household chores; and holidays spent mostly on the beach. This of course is an outline of a typical Western life-style.

As already mentioned, the process of digestion itself uses about ten per cent of the energy from food. So for example 2500 calories eaten a day require around 250 calories for digestion; 1500 calories eaten a day require 150 for digestion.

So a fair estimate of the total energy needs of a sedentary person can be produced, allowing roughly twenty-five per cent above the basic level for living and another ten per cent or thereabouts for digestion. A sedentary man of eleven stone will be in energy balance (meaning, that he will tend to stay the same weight) eating around 2400 calories from food a day. The equivalent figure for a woman of eight stone eight pounds, is around 1750 calories a day. The figures, in round terms, are:

	Rest (calories)	Digestion (calories)	Living (calories)	Total (calories)
Man (11 stone)	1700	250	450	2400
Woman (8 stone 8)	1200	200	300	1700

These figures are substantially below those recommended by the World Health Organisation for people defined as 'fairly active'. This definition covers people who take some trouble to compensate for having sedentary jobs, or people whose jobs involve them walking around a lot, such as postmen, or else who engage in regular active recreation like gardening, tennis or golf. For such people the WHO figures are around 3000 calories a day for the eleven stone man under fifty years old, and around 2200 calories a day for the equivalent eight stone eight pound woman.

The energy required by the fairly active person for all activity, including digestion, is a bit more than half as much again as that required by the body at rest. But for fairly active as well as sedentary people the energy the body requires when asleep and at rest is much greater than that required for activity.

Dieting slows you down

On a diet, the body of a fairly active person can thus accommodate a drop of a few hundred calories by becoming much less active. But the body of a sedentary person does not have so much room for manoeuvre. And in any case, diet regimes usually stipulate 1000 to 1500 calories a day or less.

How does the body accommodate such a sharp cut? The diet book theory, which might seem common sense, is that the body has no option but to lose fat. But in fact the body has many other options. And it not only takes these options so as to protect the storehouse of fat, by losing glycogen, water and lean tissue and by slowing down its waking activity. It also slows down its vital functions. The dieter's metabolic rate, like that of anyone who fasts or who is starving, slows down to adapt to the new situation.

The diet books have ignored the scientific studies of this phenomenon, although these are well known to specialists in obesity and energy balance. The fact that human metabolism is not static but dynamic, and is depressed by dieting, is such vital knowledge that it is worth going into some detail in describing the studies that have proved the point.

People who believe that dieting works have often said to me, 'but nobody ever got fat in a concentration camp'. This macabre fact is presented in support of the idea that what amounts to the voluntary semi-starvation of dieting, will reduce overweight people to some point short of emaciation. Likewise, images of skeletal people on hunger strike, or of the victims of famine, remain in the minds of Westerners who regard themselves as well fed as evidence that dieting works.

Dr Marian Apfelbaum, of the Bichat Hospital in Paris, investigated what happened to the people of the Warsaw Ghetto during the two years of famine in the Second World War. It is known that their average daily calorie intake was between 700 and 800: maybe 1700 calories a day less than they consumed before the famine.

It is safe to assume that the average weight of body fat (also known as 'adipose tissue') in an adult is about thirty pounds, representing roughly 100,000 calories. A deficit of 1700 calories a day for two years amounts to a total deficit of 1,000,000 calories, in round figures: 'approximately ten times the equivalent in energy of the adipose stores', as Apfelbaum says. What, then, happened to the remaining deficit of 900,000 calories?

A less extreme but better documented case is of 700 Swiss whose calorie intake was measured between 1942 and 1946. In 1942 the average intake was 2400 calories a day, as it was in 1946. In the intervening years, food restrictions forced the intake down to 2100 calories a day; then 2000, then 1850. The accumulated deficit, taking 2400 calories a day as the norm, was 600,000 calories per person. But the average weight loss for the whole period was twenty pounds a person which, measured as body fat, amounts to 60,000 calories. What happened to the remaining 540,000 calories?

Apfelbaum reviewed these cases of forced restriction of food because he was concerned with:

> The problem of an obese person who loses weight on a restricted diet but then stops. Physicians in the past have tended to say that such a patient must be a liar, because they considered that energy expenditure was not influenced by energy intake. I think they were wrong.

And he concluded: 'There is a wealth of evidence showing that there is a reduction in energy expenditure with restricted diet.' That is to say, dieting slows down the metabolic rate.

The classic experiments on the physiology of dieting were carried out in the USA by F G Benedict in 1919 and by Ancel Keys in 1945. Benedict put thirty-four student volunteers on a diet first of 2100, then of 1500 calories a day: as healthy young men their normal requirement was 3100 calories. The goal of the experiment was to achieve a weight loss of ten per cent, which took sixty days. But their metabolic rate declined to a greater extent than this loss of body weight could account for: by eighteen per cent.

Keys' project was more ambitious. He restricted thirty-six volunteers to a diet of 1570 calories a day but for a longer period: twenty-four weeks. The volunteers were highly motivated, being conscientious objectors who felt it appropriate to deprive themselves. At the end of twenty-four weeks their weight had on average declined by twenty-four per cent. But their metabolic rate at rest had declined by thirty-nine per cent. Like many women slimmers, these young men also damaged their health.

The outward signs of this loss of vitality were lethargy and apathy. The young men lost interest in themselves, in each other, in sex and in visitors. They stopped spontaneous play and avoided work. Two had mental breakdowns. All became obsessed with food.

Some studies, including one recently made by Dr John Garrow and co-workers of nineteen very obese women who lost an average of sixty-six pounds in a year by means of jaw-wiring, have shown a drop in resting metabolic rate matched by weight loss. But studies of people on restricted diets in less extreme circumstances, corresponding to the situation of all but the most obese dieters, consistently support the findings of Benedict and Keys: the drop in metabolic rate outmatches the drop in weight.

George Bray, Professor of Medicine at UCLA, put six overweight women on a diet of 450 calories for twenty-four days. He reported in *The Lancet* that their weight dropped by an average of twenty-two pounds, a drop of seven per cent. But their energy expenditure dropped by fifteen per cent.

Derek Miller of Queen Elizabeth College, London, Audrey Eyton's nutritional adviser, is a campaigner against the notion that, as he puts it, obesity is caused by 'either or both of the deadly sins, gluttony and sloth'. He is clear that 'energy intake and expenditure influence each other'.

Like Apfelbaum, Miller contradicts the notion that dieters who say that they eat little are lying. He took thirty veteran dieters from slimming clubs to Ragdale Hall, an isolated country house. Their luggage was searched, their car keys taken away, and they were fed a diet supplying the same number of calories as Benedict and Keys gave their young male volunteers: 1500 a day. Miller's regime lasted for three weeks. The metabolic rate of these seasoned dieters was so low that 'although nineteen subjects lost weight, nine maintained within plus or minus a kilogram (2.2 pounds), and two actually gained weight'.

Derek Miller believes that he is now hot on the trail of what, for some, might prove the richest prize in obesity research: a drug to speed up the metabolic rate, which can be patented. It is safe to predict that a drug firm will soon announce that it is putting an anti-fat pill on the market. The two most common methods used currently to speed up the metabolic rate, are smoking and amphetamines; both addictive, and more damaging to health than obesity. Doctors I have spoken to believe that there is no such thing as a safe drug that speeds up the metabolic rate.

Meanwhile, a famous statement made by Professor Albert Stunkard, of the University of Pennsylvania, still holds good:

> Most obese people do not enter treatment for obesity. Of those who do enter, most will not remain. Of those who remain, most will not lose much weight. Of those who lose weight, most will regain it.

The dangers of dieting

What mechanism does the body use to slow its metabolic rate? The most efficient would be to slow the function of the body's most metabolically active cells: those in the vital organs. The dramatic drop in metabolic rate produced by these experiments cannot be because of loss of fat, because fat is a relatively inactive part of the body. Ancel Keys proposes a mechanism that might well give any dieter pause for thought:

> It appears that the tissue loss and the changes in the metabolic rate of the liver and other organs with high metabolic rate may be of considerable importance in explaining the changes in basal metabolism during starvation and food restriction.

And he calculates that eighty per cent of the decrease in oxygen consumption in his subjects can be accounted for by a halving of the oxygen used by the liver and its associated organs.

The body needs oxygen all the time for its vital functions. The greater the body's capacity for oxygen, the fitter a person will be. A high capacity for oxygen protects against diseases of the heart, lungs and blood vessels. But the consequence of dieting, Keys proposes, is dramatically to lower the body's use of oxygen. Dieting cannot in itself be a healthy activity.

Dr Apfelbaum recently reviewed the results obtained in twenty-four studies of under-nutrition made between 1903 and 1969. Men and women of widely varying weight and in different circumstances were underfed for different reasons for periods varying between three weeks and two years. The amount of energy consumed as food in these studies ranged from 1600 calories a day to 700 – 1200 (several) to zero – fasting. 'All the authors report a decrease of the basal metabolic rate as a result of diet restriction ranging from ten to forty-five per cent according to the length and stringency of the restriction.'

Professor Stunkard confirms that dieting slows down the metabolic rate and frustrates the dieter. He goes on to say: 'Repeated attempts at weight reduction may lead to a progressive slowing of weight loss and to even more rapid regaining of weight.'

I have yet to read of any account of this phenomenon in any diet book. This is not surprising. The facts that the scientists have known for decades, and that have been set down in scientific journals and textbooks, make most diet books so much waste paper.

Now, in 1983, the British medical establishment is acknowledging that metabolism is dynamic. The Royal College of Physicians, referring to some of the studies summarised here, put a bomb under the diet books by saying, in their report on obesity:

> It has been known for many years that there are substantial differences in the metabolic rates of individuals at rest and also that the body is able to adapt to changes in energy intake. If volunteers are given only half their usual intake, there is an early fall in the metabolic rate of the tissues.

Dieting slows you down more than weight loss can explain because dieting slows down the processes of the most active vital organs in the body. This process can be dangerous if the diet is extreme or prolonged or unbalanced, or if the dieter is not in good health, or if the dieting is repeated over a number of years. Millions of people, women mostly, in Great Britain, the USA and other countries go in for fad diets every year. They are damaging their health.

The more severe the diet, the more you slow down. Fasting has the most dramatic effect. 'Energy requirements decrease by twenty-five to thirty per cent in the course of three to four weeks of fasting,' reports Ernst Drenick, an American doctor who favours fasting as a treatment for obese patients. He goes on to say:

> Restraint should be advised in the amounts of food allowed after fasting or after the desired weight level has been attained with fasting. The adaptive lowering of the metabolic rate may quickly lead to substantial weight gains if normal, average meals are consumed during this period.

In other words, the only way not to put on the weight that has been lost by fasting is to go on a diet after the fast has ended.

Fasting wastes muscle

Drenick subjected 137 very fat people to fasts of between one and four months. The average weight loss was sixty-four pounds. The patients were well pleased. However, when 105 were followed up two years later, ninety-six had regained their pre-fast weight. Drenick acknowledges that during two-month fasts his subjects lost seventeen pounds of muscle on average, but he does not suggest that this is why they regained weight. Instead, he says that 'regular revisits and close supervision' during the follow-up period are crucial and concludes:

> Our experiences are disappointing. [But] a sizeable number of the subjects had been on welfare for years; many of them had never been usefully employed. Therefore solid motivation over the long run might be questioned in some of these patients.

In other words, the experiment is valid, but the subjects are not up to standard – a new version of 'the operation was successful, but the patient died.' Sometimes, fasting results in death from heart failure. So does fasting modified by the administration of liquid protein, a regime made popular in America by Robert Linn's book *The Last Chance Diet.* In 1978 the American government investigated fifty-eight cases in which this liquid protein diet had led to death from heart failure. The more extreme a diet is, the more dangerous it is.

But what happens to patients who do survive fasts? Frederick Benoit, a Californian doctor, subjected seven fat US naval personnel to a fast quick enough to tempt impatient dieters: ten days. In this time the average weight lost was just over twenty pounds. However: 'the mean weight loss from fasting was due to 64.6 per cent decrease in lean body weight and only 35.4 per cent loss in body fat.' Benoit concludes 'fasting beyond ten days may produce decreasing rates of lean tissue breakdown' but 'the wisdom of incurring such wastes in lean body tissue is open to question'.

There is something to be said for fasting. People who occasionally fast for a day or two often find the experience refreshing. But fasting is not a way to lose fat. It slows down the body's activity dramatically, to a point as close as ordinary people ever get to hibernation, and it wastes lean body tissue, including muscle, designed to be metabolically active. Fasting changes the composition of the body, so that after the fast the body works at a lower energy level than before it started, not only because weight has been lost but also because of the wasting of metabolically active tissue. Special exercises, like those used by physiotherapists to rehabilitate people whose muscles have been wasted as a result of inactivity after a surgical operation, are the only way to restore the body to its previous metabolic rate after it has undergone a prolonged fast.

Over-eating speeds you up

If dieting slows you down, and fasting slows you down even more, does it follow that over-feeding will speed up the metabolic rate? Yes, it does. Over-feeding does not make you thin, of course, but it does speed up the rate at which the body uses energy. The studies on this subject are as extensive as those on under-feeding.

In 1901, a German, R O Neumann, reported the results of an experiment upon himself, in which he over-ate for long periods. After an initial weight gain, he found that he could eat 800 calories a day above his normal intake and gain little extra weight. His conclusion was that 'someone who is healthy can take in surplus food and consume it by burning it faster.'

This experiment was repeated by Derek Miller in the 1960s, when forty-nine subjects were encouraged to eat at least 1000 calories a day above their normal intake for periods of up to eight weeks:

> There was a marked weekly adaptation to the calorie load, such that the rate of weight gain fell throughout the experiment. There was a marked individual variation, and it is quite remarkable how some individuals can eat an excess of 10,000 calories a week and show a weight loss.

After over-feeding, a person's metabolic rate when asleep and at rest speeds up, as does the energy given off as a direct result of eating. Most remarkable of all is the effect on the energy used when exercising. In one study the oxygen consumed by people who were over-eating increased by thirty per cent during walking, twenty-five per cent during cycling and nineteen per cent during stair-climbing. Oxygen consumed during exercise is a measure of energy used. By contrast, Ernst Drenick found that after a three- to seven-week fast, oxygen consumption decreased by twenty-one per cent during bed rest, thirty-two per cent when sitting, and forty per cent when walking. The human body will always adapt to circumstances, and seek balance.

Diets train the body to adapt to the circumstances of dieting, which it does by slowing down its vital functions. This adaptive behaviour is the best means of staying alive and as healthy as possible in famine. As already stated, our minds know the difference between going on a diet and famine or starvation; but our bodies do not.

Different people, different speeds

Different people have different metabolic rates, for a variety of factors that help to explain why some people never get fat and other people get fat very easily. These include physical make-up, mental state, the circumstances in which people live, and their state of health; how active they are; and how fit they are. Some of these factors cannot be altered, others can be. Not only is metabolism dynamic, slowing down or speeding up according to the volume of food eaten; it is also variable at will. Dieters feel imprisoned in their bodies partly because they do not realise that they can speed up their metabolic rate. Within wide limits we can choose how much energy we want our bodies to use; it is literally a question of how lively we choose to be.

Other things being equal, a heavy person needs more energy than a light person. Someone who loses weight will use less energy and need less food simply because of being lighter. A tall person needs more energy than a short person because a larger body surface enables more heat to escape.

Because body fat is metabolically less active than fat-free tissue – muscle and the vital organs in particular – the greater the proportion of fat-free tissue in the body, the more therefore the energy requirement. Similarly, the greater the proportion of fat in the body, the less energy that is required. This means that other things being equal, a lean person needs more energy from food, and uses more energy from oxygen, than does a fat person. Fat people can have metabolic rates higher than thin people because of being heavier altogether, and having bigger bodies with more fat-free tissue, notwithstanding having a lot of fat. Weight for weight, though, lean people are likely to have relatively high metabolic rates because of being lean; fat people are likely to have relatively low metabolic rates because of being fat.

Men are usually not only heavier and taller than women, but also usually have less body fat. The average woman has around nine per cent more body fat than the average man. There are three types of body fat: subcutaneous, deposited under the skin; depot, lying deeper, characteristically on the belly in men and around the hips and thighs in women; and essential fat, within the body to protect the vital organs. Women have more depot and essential body fat than men. The average man uses more energy than the average woman, not because he is a man (whatever that might mean) but because he is heavier, taller and leaner. A woman and man of the same height, weight and body composition will have the same energy requirements.

Energy breeds energy

From adulthood onwards, energy requirements decline by about five per cent a decade. It follows that the average sixty-year-old requires about twenty per cent less food than the average twenty-year-old. The World Health Organisation's recommended figures for daily energy intake from food are:

age	men (11 st) (calories)	women (8 st 8 lb) (calories)
16 – 19	3600	2400
20 – 29	3200	2300
30 – 39	3100	2200
40 – 49	3000	2200
50 – 59	2800	2000
60 – 69	2500	1800
70 +	2200	1600

It is true that maximum oxygen capacity, a measure of physical energy requirement, declines slowly as a function of age, at a rate of about two per cent a decade. But these figures mostly reflect the fact that what exercise young people in the West do take, declines almost to zero in middle age. People who remain active into old age continue to need, and to use, high amounts of energy. Elderly Swiss farmers of both sexes have been observed to have an energy requirement as high as 4000 to 5000 calories a day.

The sedentary man or woman who becomes less active but eats more in middle age is in trouble. Having said that the significance of physical activity in weight gain in middle age has up to now been under-emphasised, the Royal College of Physicians report on obesity states:

increasing inactivity in middle age forms the basis for the decline in muscle mass and lean body mass as people grow older. The replacement of lean tissue by fat with ageing compounds the problem of energy balance, since the basal

45

need for energy falls with the reduction in metabolically active lean tissue; this will lead to a further drop in the basal metabolic rate and a tendency to gain body fat.

As a rule, adolescents require more energy than adults, for their growth as well as their activity. Pregnant women need about 300 extra calories a day; lactating women, about 500 extra calories a day.

A very small number of people suffer from a disorder of their metabolic function and become grossly obese despite eating normal amounts of food. These people do indeed have 'something wrong with their glands'. A number of the patients hospitalised in obesity wards are dangerously overweight for such reasons and, simply because they are available to doctors, have been much studied. Without treatment of the underlying cause of their obesity, not much can be done for them long-term by diet regimes.

Recent work done by Dr Michael Stock and Nancy Rothwell in London indicates that a special type of body fat, brown fat, present in small but variable quantities at various sites in the body, is very active metabolically. Most of the work done on brown fat has been carried out on rats, and it is not yet known whether we can increase our brown fat stores and so burn energy faster.

To say that people have a high metabolic rate is to say, in scientific terms, that they use a lot of energy. An energetic person uses those parts of the body that are metabolically active and will therefore need and use more energy at rest and when active. Diet books discourage us from taking account of what, given reflection and self-awareness, we already know: energy breeds energy.

Mental and emotional states, and physical health, also affect the speed at which our bodies work. Being 'high' or 'low' is not just a mental state; it reflects high or low biochemical states. Elation and fever are two examples of high states, one good, one bad; both require and use more energy. Depression literally depresses the body's energy. People who feel low may gain fat not because they eat

46

more food but because the food they are eating, normally the right amount, is too much in a depressed state. Depressed people who worry about weight but are unaware that depression affects the rate at which the body uses energy are in a vicious circle. Lacking guidance, they are liable to eat a normal amount of food, gain fat, and so become more depressed. If a pattern is established, the result may be self-destructive behaviour, such as eating abnormally large quantities of food, ('bingeing').

People in industrialised societies have lost touch with their bodies. But animals that become out of sorts or physically depressed, for whatever reason, spend a lot of time resting and sleeping. So do people in tribal societies. The body has its own energy resources. Pressing food on someone who is ill is usually completely the wrong thing to do; the body's energy needs to be directed to the source of the illness, not to digestion.

Lean people use most energy

The common experience of one particularly strong emotion, the state of 'being in love', is that the lover refuses food when he or she is secretly pining after the loved one. If Romeo and Juliet wanted to lose weight in the first part of their play, they were in luck. But if love has the lineaments of gratified desire and is altogether active, not passive, then the Tom Jones syndrome applies, and the lover is liable to eat with the appetite of the furnace of a steam locomotive.

This account of the physical, mental and emotional circumstances that determine and change metabolic rate, and also of the amount of energy the body needs and uses, is really nothing more than common sense. Dieting depresses the human organism. And the mental depression that follows dieting is caused by this physical depression. Dieting slows down the spirit as well as the body. Christian evangelists preach the mortification of the flesh as the only means to achieve grace. Diet books substitute health for faith but otherwise use the same

47

techniques. And the promises made by diet books are illusions.

The more you weigh, and the more lean body tissue you have, the higher metabolic rate will tend to be at all times – when asleep, when resting and when active.

The tables of energy requirements from food, such as those published by the World Health Organisation and in books of nutrition, give body weight, together with age, as the only factors affecting resting metabolic rate (that is, the speed at which the body works at complete rest, just after sleep). In one crucial respect these tables are misleading. They imply that heavy people have a high metabolic rate and so require more food simply because they are heavy; and that light people, likewise, have a low metabolic rate and so require less food simply because they are light. And this is only half of the story.

What dieters, and by contrast very active people, especially need to know is that the people who have the lowest metabolic rate are people who, as well as being light, are also fat; and that the people who have the highest metabolic rate are people who, as well as being heavy, are also lean. Of course, it is true that, more often than not, light people are lean and heavy people are fat. But this is not the case for very many people in Western countries. A tall male manual worker may be a muscular, lean fourteen stone. A middle-aged sedentary woman may be no more than eight stone but, if she is no more than average height, be very flabby; that is to say, have little lean tissue and much fat on her body.

It follows that a light, lean person can have the same metabolic rate as a heavy, fat person. Professor John Durnin has calculated that it is possible for a lean person weighing eight stone to need and use the same amount of energy as a fat person weighing eleven stone. The table opposite is re-calculated from Professor Durnin's book *Energy, Work and Leisure*, and shows, in round figures, the amount of resting energy needed per day by people not only of different weights, but also of different body compositions.

Resting metabolic rates of men and women of different weight and body composition

Men	Women	8 stone (cals)	9½ stone (cals)	11 stone (cals)	12½ stone (cals)	14 stone (cals)
Lean		1450	1650	1850	2050	2250
Average	Lean	1300	1500	1700	1900	2100
Fat	Average	1150	1350	1550	1750	1950
Obese	Fat	1000	1200	1400	1600	1800
	Obese	850	1050	1250	1450	1650

In this table, an 'average' man is equivalent to a 'lean' woman because, as stated, women have more body fat than men. Thus, a lean man has around ten per cent total body fat; a lean woman, around twenty per cent. Likewise, a 'fat' man, as here defined, has about thirty per cent body fat; a 'fat' woman, about forty per cent.

So, what these figures show, is that (to take extreme cases) a fat person of eight stone (the short-ish middle-aged woman) has a resting requirement of 1000 calories of food a day; a lean person of fourteen stone (the tall manual worker) requires 2250 calories of food a day. Now, assume that the woman is sedentary, but not unusually so, and uses twenty-five per cent above her resting metabolic rate for activity. Also assume that the man uses 1800 calories of energy a day because of his work (which is roughly accurate if he is working fairly vigorously for six hours a day). The figures, in round terms, come out as follows:

	Rest (calories)	Digestion (calories)	Living (calories)	Total (calories)
Lean man (14 stone)	2250	450	1800	4000
Fat woman (8 stone)	1000	150	250	1400

Thanks to Professor Durnin's calculations, it is now clear why an active man can, indeed, 'eat like a horse' and yet stay lean, while an inactive woman can, indeed, 'eat like a bird' and yet gain weight and fat. The figures show why

49

Derek Miller's experiment had the result that it did; for 1500 calories a day can be over the top, for some women.

What these figures also show, is that a big, active person can take more liberties with food, than can a small, inactive person. Keeping with the examples above, the fat eight stone woman will be eating more than twice her daily energy requirement for the life she leads, if she eats a couple of slices of cake, or four digestive biscuits, over the odds. Indeed, the same applies to a young woman who drinks an extra orange juice and also an extra soft drink in one day. By contrast, the lean fourteen stone man can have six extra twelve-ounce cans of beer and yet be consuming only half as much again as he normally requires. All he needs to do, to get back in energy balance, is to lay off the chips for a couple of days, or else to go for a run.

The people who are most unfortunate of all, are women who have put themselves through diet regime after diet regime, throughout their adult lives. As a result they will slowly but surely have wasted their metabolically active lean tissue; they will have lost the ability to take exercise; and they will, quite likely, be artificially light yet artificially fat, because of the futile misery they have put themselves through. Such women could literally be obese weighing only nine and a half stone and, literally, slowly gain fat eating no more than 1500 calories a day. It is impossible for such a woman to be healthy, for reasons explained in the next chapter ('Sugar Makes You Hungry'). The writers of diet books bear a heavy responsibility.

An inactive woman of eight stone cannot transform herself into an active man of fourteen stone. But, sticking with the same example, suppose a fat, inactive woman of eight stone became a lean, active woman of eight stone, choosing a new life which involved an extra 750 calories of energy a day in exercise? How would the sums look, then?

	Rest (calories)	Digestion (calories)	Living (calories)	Total (calories)
Fat woman (8 stone)	1000	150	250	1400
Lean woman (8 stone)	1300	250	1000	2550

Weight for weight, a lean woman can eat 1000 calories a day more than a fat woman. The taller and heavier the woman, the greater the contrast. And here is the answer to the diet books. Active people can eat the equivalent of a meal a day more than inactive people, and stay lean while the inactive people continue to get fat.

Fat regained

If a fat woman of, say, eleven stone could, by dieting, reduce to eight stone, and if the diet worked according to her dream, so that all the weight lost was fat, then she could eat almost as much food at the lean weight of eight stone as she previously did at the fat weight of eleven stone. But this dream is a fantasy which – as most dieters know – is liable to become a waking nightmare.

As a rule, any diet that has resulted in a loss of ten or fifteen pounds in the first week or three, will result in a gain of the same amount in a month or so after the diet has ended. A crash diet lasting a few days that results in a loss of, say, six pounds, will result in that weight being regained just as fast, if not faster.

The reason, as explained, is that diets drain glycogen and water, and after a diet this glycogen and water is bound to be replaced. Typically, writers of diet books make dieters believe that weight lost is of fat, and weight regained is because of greed. It is time that doctors and dieters knew that the diet books are wrong.

It is of course true that any diet prolonged over a period of weeks will result in a loss of fat, together with glycogen and water, and metabolically active lean tissue. But the loss of non-fat tissue has the effect of artificially lowering the body's energy requirements.

If a dieter is prepared to follow a prolonged diet with what is in effect a modified diet for life, then, indeed, it is possible to keep lost weight off. Millions of women in the West do just that. The cost is depression, weakness, exhaustion and permanent malnutrition caused by deprivation of the food a body needs to be healthy. Again, if, after a diet, lighter people become a lot more active, maybe because of liking the look of the new physical self, then they can not only keep lost fat off, but also eat more and at the same time become leaner. The reasons are fully explained in a later chapter ('More Air! More Air!') The happy people who become active after a diet, become slim not because of the diet but because they follow their diet with exercise. The only people I know who have kept much weight off in the long term after a diet has ended are those who started to exercise regularly during or after the diet.

The fact is, that most people regain the weight lost on a diet. In her book *Fat is a Feminist Issue*, Susie Orbach claims that in the long term ninety-five per cent of all dieters regain all the weight lost on diet regimes. This figure, which is quite often quoted, is open to doubt. But it is safe to say that the eventual result of dieting is as likely to be a net weight gain as a net weight loss. The Royal College of Physicians report on obesity states:

> Maintenance of weight loss beyond one year was less satisfactory and all longer-term studies have found that weight increases again in the majority of patients. In the most complete study, 154 of the 190 patients who had been treated one to five years previously were found for questioning. Twenty-five (sixteen per cent) had maintained a weight loss of over forty pounds and twenty-seven (seventeen per cent) were heavier than at the start of the study.

Weightwatchers, and *Slimming* magazine (founded and then published by Audrey Eyton of *The F-Plan Diet*) promote newspaper and magazine features, and publish books, graphically showing massive weight loss of slimmers who have used their methods. Commercial slimming clubs are not, however, noted for long-term follow-up studies. Nor, it must be said, are doctors. In 1979 Rena Wing and Robert Jeffery of the University of Pittsburgh Medical School completed a review of 145 slimming projects involving 6927 patients, published between 1966 and 1977 with medical supervision. Of these, eight only included a follow-up one year or more after the project was 'complete'. Indeed, only forty-three included a follow-up of any duration at all. The reason, of course, is that diet regimes do not work, and that people responsible for the administration of diet regimes do not want to admit to themselves, and certainly not to the overweight people who come to them, that the treatment will almost certainly fail. Like football pools promoters, slimming clubs advertise their rare winners.

Very few people indeed eat sparingly immediately after a diet has ended. Almost invariably they respond to the body's cravings by eating at least as much as they ate before the diet started. This is not because of habit, nor, however much the dieters may blame themselves, because of greed, stupidity or thoughtlessness. The body needs energy to regenerate and responds to the first days after a diet has ended with signals of extreme hunger.

And woe to the sedentary dieter. Once the glycogen and water has been replaced, the body of the sedentary person, being used to fat, will tend to regain fat and will rebuild less muscle, simply because muscle is used less by an inactive person. For a sedentary person the result of a diet, once weight has been regained after it has ended, is to alter the composition of the body. The proportion of lean tissue in the body decreases; the proportion of fatty tissue increases. Muscle is lost; fat is gained. This is one of the reasons why dieting makes you fat.

Nobody ever became fat in a concentration camp. But the survivors of concentration camps who resumed sedentary lives did tend to become fat. Prison camp diets devastate muscle. The people who survived Hitler's death camps frequently became very flabby after the war; not necessarily heavy, but fat.

The consequences of a single diet regime, even if severe and prolonged, for a sedentary person, need not be damaging. The change in composition of the body after one diet is unlikely to be dramatic. All the same, Dr Garrow's comment on Benedict's sixty-day and Keys' twenty-four-week experiments is a warning to any optimist willing to trust to willpower:

> It is interesting that the volunteers for the semi-starvation experiments of Benedict et al (1919) and Keys et al (1950) tended to over-eat and become obese after the termination of the experiment.

In both cases 'semi-starvation' consisted of regimes of 1500 calories a day. After his experiment was over, Keys put his subjects on a gradual re-feeding programme, of the kind all diet books recommend as sensible. The men remained ravenous. After the re-feeding programme ended and the men could eat as much as they liked, some became ill from over-eating; they averaged a consumption of 5000 calories a day; and regained their pre-diet weights without regaining all their muscle tissue. They began slim, they ended obese.

Energy lost

For a sedentary person a lifetime spent between diets is not only self-defeating but also dangerous. Every diet trains the body to adapt to dieting, which it does by slowing itself down, losing some lean tissue and not replacing all of it. Every diet alters the composition of the body cumulatively.

Dieting makes you fat because of this cumulative change in the composition of the body. A second reason why dieting makes you fat is that fat is lighter than muscle. The net result of a diet, for a sedentary person, may be a loss of weight. But the body of such a dieter may nevertheless contain a greater proportion of fat. Certainly any sedentary dieter who regains the weight lost after a diet is bound to be fatter than when the diet started, simply because they will have replaced heavier muscle with lighter and bulkier fat.

A third reason why dieting makes you fat is because fat is less metabolically active than muscle. The greater the proportion of fat in the body, the lower the metabolic rate of that body and, therefore, the less energy required from food. Paradoxically, this process is a sign that the body is functioning efficiently; the most self-protective reaction the body can have to a diet regime, to which it reacts as if to a state of famine, is to adapt the better to survive the next famine. This it does best by requiring less food and by storing more fat.

For a sedentary person, the one sure way to slow the body down and so create the conditions for getting fat is to go on a diet. Every diet trains the body to become less energetic, to require less energy from food, and to use less energy from oxygen with which to burn food. Habitual dieters are on a downward spiral which remorselessly reduces their vitality.

This is why dieting makes you fat.

But why does up to half the population of Great Britain, the USA and other industrialised societies steadily gain weight and fat throughout life? Why do we get fat in the first place?

CHAPTER THREE

Sugar Makes You Hungry

The aspects of things that are most important for us are
hidden because of their simplicity and familiarity. One is
unable to notice something – because it is always before
one's eyes. We fail to be struck by what, once seen, is most
striking and most powerful.
LUDWIG WITTGENSTEIN
Philosophical Investigations

Breathing at my side, that heavy animal,
That heavy bear that sleeps with me,
Howls in his sleep for a world of sugar,
A sweetness intimate as the water's clasp.
DELMORE SCHWARTZ
The Heavy Bear That Goes With Me

Why do we get fat?

For every dieter there's another man or woman who
doesn't diet but who gets fat all the same. Nobody wants
to be fat. Yet most people over the age of thirty in Great
Britain, the USA and other countries will acknowledge
that they'd like to lose some weight (meaning, fat, of
course). That is why diet books have such massive sales.

Every year scores of millions of people in the West go
on diets; which don't work. Scores of millions more
people get fat without going on diets. People in
industrialised societies have tended to get fatter and fatter
during this century. The trend is continuing. A year never
goes by without a representative body of scientists or
doctors in the USA or Great Britain stating, again, that
obesity is a massive public health problem. An American

team of experts with a sense of humour recently worked out that the US adult population was carrying a total of 2297 million pounds of excess fat which, if converted into energy, would be enough to supply the annual residential electricity demands of Boston, Chicago, San Francisco and Washington.

It was not always so. Dieting is almost entirely a twentieth-century phenomenon. One hundred years ago and more, few people dieted – because they didn't need to. Few, other than the rich (whose faces are commemorated in paintings) and dandies like Byron, tended to get fat. And dieting is almost entirely a Western phenomenon. There still are very many millions of people in the world living away from Western influence – hunter-gatherers, pastoralists, farmers, peasants and people in remote countries – who may eat well, live to a ripe old age, but do not tend to gain weight and get fat as they get older. In the Third World it is only when people move from the countryside to the towns, or when they start to eat Western-influenced food, that they put on fat. It is the rich (whose pictures we see in the papers and on television) who most commonly get fat.

Diet books and most obesity textbooks assume that we get fat because we are eating more and more. Some people of course do get fat because they eat great quantities of food. But greed is not the usual reason. Overall, people in the West are eating less and less while becoming fatter and fatter. What, then, can be the cause of our overweight?

The massive difference between the food we in the West eat and the food eaten by everyone until this century is a difference primarily not of quantity, but of quality. Measured in the conventional way, we eat about the same amount of protein as do people in the Third World who live in settled societies; rather less carbohydrate; and a great deal more fat. The most impressive difference, though, is between whole food and processed food. In particular, all studies made of the differences between the foods eaten in Western and non-Western societies show that people in the West eat great amounts of processed carbohydrate, sugar especially; whereas people who live away from Western influence, including people in Western countries which are little influenced by industrialisation, eat great amounts of whole carbohydrate, starch especially. And people in the West get fat, whereas, as a rule, non-Western people do not.

It makes sense to discover whether the connection between processed carbohydrates, sugar in particular, and fatness is causal or merely coincidental.

The rise of the sweet tooth

Until recently sugar was a luxury. In 1300 AD a pound of sugar cost a year's pay; it was then a chic item on the tables of the cosmopolitan rich, much as cocaine is today. In 1700, Great Britain was importing twenty million pounds of sugar a year; in 1800, 160 million pounds. Sugar was of course the main non-human commodity of the slave trade, which helped to make Great Britain the richest and most powerful nation in the world. By 1850 consumption of sugar had risen to about twenty pounds a person a year. The tax on sugar helped to pay for the Crimean War. In 1874 Gladstone removed the tax on sugar, and consumption rose steeply, so that in 1900 every man, woman and child in Great Britain was eating an average of seventy-two pounds of processed sugar a year, and expenditure on sugar matched that on bread. The British sweet tooth was bred a century ago, and it was then that sweet foods became popular in shops and at home.

Consumption of sugar continued to rise during this century, except during the two world wars. By the mid-1950s, with sweets and confectionery off the ration again, the British were eating more sugar than ever before. For the last thirty years the volume of sugar manufactured in and imported to Great Britain has been of the order of 2,500,000 tons a year, or around 100 pounds for every man, woman and child.

In the financial year 1981 the British Sugar Corporation turned over £488,200,000, and made a profit of £51,035,000. Projected profits for 1982 were £64 million.

(The term 'sugar' here, means processed white and brown sugar, commonly known as 'refined' sugar. I use the term 'processed sugar' for manufactured sugar which has no nourishment in it, in contrast to natural sugar in whole fruit and vegetables which are nutritious.)

The average consumption of processed sugar in Great Britain is therefore about two pounds a week, a head. On average, sedentary people in Britain consume around twenty per cent of their energy in the form of processed sugar.

The world average consumption of processed sugar is now about one-third of the British figure. The overall African figure is about one-fifth, but is rising. The overall Asian figure is about one-eighth, but is also rising. Wherever Coca-Cola signs can be found, more and more sugar is being eaten.

There was a time when the British ate more sugar than any other nation; that time has now passed. People in Mediterranean countries still eat less of it; but 100 pounds a year is, as a round figure, accurate for North America, Western Europe and other developed countries.

In Great Britain about two-thirds of all sugar eaten is contained within manufactured food, and of this well over half is in chocolate, confectionery, cakes, biscuits and soft drinks. Chocolate is over half sugar; sweets are almost all sugar; a Mars Bar, the most popular British confectionery line, is nearly sixty-six per cent sugar; biscuits vary between ten and forty-five per cent sugar; soft drinks such as Coca-Cola are about ninety per cent water and ten per cent sugar.

Some people eat less, some more, than the average of 100 pounds a year of sugar. Adolescents and young men and women without the means or inclination to prepare or buy their own meals, who snack a lot, may eat 200 pounds a year, or even more; a figure approaching half their energy requirement from food.

To someone without a sweet tooth the figure of 100 pounds a year, which includes only processed, 'refined', sugar but not natural sugars in fruit and some vegetables, may seem remarkably high. But sugar is used very extensively by food manufacturers.

Some foods regarded as healthy, or at least not thought of as sweet, contain a lot of processed sugar, as the table 'Sugar in Food' on pages 103 – 5 shows. Sweet pickle is about one-third sugar. Canned fruits with syrup total about one-quarter sugar; as do tomato ketchup and packet muesli. Flavoured and fruit yoghurt is between thirteen and eighteen per cent sugar; baked beans are over five per cent sugar. Varying amounts of sugar are added to soups; diluted with an equal amount of water, condensed cream of tomato soup is over five per cent sugar. Anyone who wants to avoid eating processed sugar has to be alert.

In Great Britain and the USA there is now a trend towards eating less sugar at home, but more away from home. In Great Britain, Mars Bars were first manufactured in 1932. Fifty years later, 700 million were sold. Between 1932 and 1982 the amount of confectionery eaten per head went up from five and a half ounces to eight ounces a week – the extra two and a half ounces being the weight of one Mars Bar, which contains a total of 320 calories of energy.

Processed sugar is inert. It contains no vitamins and only the faintest traces of some other nutrients. In this, alone of all the foods we consume in any quantity, it is comparable only with alcoholic spirits. It supplies dead, or empty, energy. And the very last food that is suitable for a basically sedentary population is food that supplies nothing but energy. Almost all brown sugar also contains no nourishment. Sugar accurately labelled 'raw cane' sugar has some nourishment remaining.

We have been taught that the principal requirement of the human body is for quantity: readily measurable energy. This is wrong. Our principal requirement is for quality: hard-to-measure nourishment. And sugar, alone among all the substances we eat, has been processed so thoroughly that it has no nutritive value.

The advertisements of manufacturers of products sweetened by sugar foster the notion that the energy in food is used mostly for activity. This is not true. As stated in the last chapter, the lightly active person, who compensates for a sedentary job by walking, gardening, golf or other regular weekend and holiday activity, uses only one-third of the energy supplied by food for activity; the other two-thirds go to fuel the body's basic functions, and digestion. And our body needs nourishment from vitamins, minerals and other nutrients, not merely energy.

Throughout this century people in the West have

60

become less active. The car has replaced walking. Machines do housework and gardening. Much work on the farm, in factories and on building sites has been automated. People even buy electric carving knives. And yet, at the same time, more and more of the food we eat has nourishment processed out of it; and, in the case of processed sugar, has no nourishment in it at all.

Low energy, poor nourishment

I asked Arvid Wretlind about the consequences of this. Professor Wretlind, a world authority on vitamins, works for the National Institute of Public Health in Stockholm and has made a special study of the nutrition problems of people who consume small amounts of food.

He pointed out that the nutritional requirements of men and women from vitamins and minerals correspond to pre-twentieth-century energy levels. Until this century, people obtained nourishment from food supplying 2500 to 3000 calories a day or more, because their regular physical activity required a calorie intake at that level. Wretlind explains:

> The lower the physical activity the higher will be the content of the essential nutrients required per calorie in order to obtain the desired, optimal, nutritional level. A diet which is adequate for a man with a calorie requirement of 3000 calories a day cannot simply be assumed to cover the desirable nutritional supply for a low calorie consumer – for example, a woman with a calorie requirement of less than 2000 calories a day.

That is to say, people with a low energy intake need to eat especially nutritious food to have any chance of getting enough vitamins and minerals. Studies show that varying groups of people with a low energy intake receive insufficient nutrients, for example vitamin A (carotene), riboflavin (vitamin B2), vitamin C (ascorbic acid), calcium and iron. Wretlind's conclusion is that:

> The low caloric group, such as schoolgirls, office girls, women, and old-age pensioners do not receive a supply of

nutrients corresponding to that considered desirable for good nutritional conditions.

Here he is describing healthy people of normal habits; or, at least, superficially healthy people, for he goes on to say that in Western countries, 'a number of disturbances occur in the state of health and well-being which are either wholly or partially due to the unsuitable composition of the diet or to defective dietary habits'.

When you think about it, this view is common sense. Take an average-size woman who, before this century, would have been in energy balance eating nourishing food with an energy value of say 2500 calories. The equivalent woman of the same height now, who has an office job, will be in energy balance at about 2000 calories a day, even if she takes a little exercise. Already, therefore, she can only be getting eighty per cent of the nourishment her body needs.

Now assume she is eating an average amount of processed sugar, supplying, say, 500 calories daily. It follows that she cannot be consuming more than 1500 nourishing calories daily. She is therefore getting at most, only sixty per cent of the nourishment her body needs. I would call that a state of mild chronic malnutrition, suffered not only by sedentary women but by men with office jobs, too.

Processed sugar is not, though, the only food we eat that is short of nourishment. The process of milling white flour from whole grain results in white bread that is robbed of most of the vitamins and minerals naturally present in wheat. The same applies to white rice and to any pasta that is not wholewheat. ('Brown', 'Granary' and 'wheatmeal' bread are not much better than white bread. Some 'brown' bread is not much more than coloured white bread. Good bread is 'wholewheat' or 'wholemeal').

Worse still, we in the West eat an average of forty to forty-two per cent of our calories in the form of fat, compared with the thirty per cent that was the average around the turn of the century. The body needs fat; but far less than the amount we eat. Peasant communities in the Third World do well enough eating around twelve per cent of their calories as fat. We in the West not only eat far too much fat, but also eat much animal and other saturated fats in the form of convenience food which, like white bread, is drained of nourishment. In moderation, for example, butter fresh from the farm is a healthy food. Butter 'blended' using heat, with additives, and then stored in a butter mountain for longer than the consumer can imagine, is not healthy food. Refrigerated, fats remain eatable – just – for a long time. But in that time much of what nourishment remains after the process of manufacture, disappears.

The ideal food commodity is cheap, easily transported, does not rot, preserves other foods and is highly palatable. Food is processed not in order to be more nourishing but in order to become a better commodity; to make more money. It is not by chance that Great Britain became the richest nation on earth partly by means of the profits from sugar. All manufactured foods lose nourishment. Any food advertised as having vitamins and minerals added is usually food which has lost vitamins and minerals in the process of manufacture.

We get fat in order to stay healthy

Yet more nutrients are lost in the process of preparation and cooking. Generally speaking, the more sophisticated these processes, the more nourishment is lost. (The original meaning of 'sophistication' was 'adulteration'. Brewers in previous centuries who 'sophisticated' their beer with sugar were fined or beaten.) Japanese food, celebrated as among the most healthy in the world, is undercooked. We in the West discard much of the most nutritious parts of food – skin, peel, pith from fruit and vegetables, blood and guts from meat. Then we overcook what we choose to eat, with the result that the water-soluble vitamins B and C go down the drain and many other nutrients go up in smoke.

So, the food we eat is depleted of vitamins and minerals. Processed sugar is devoid of nourishment; and processed, white – and brown – bread is short of nourishment. More nourishment in food is lost by the process of manufacture, storage, cooking, and because we discard nutritious parts of food.

We in the West are starved of vitamins for another series of reasons, also. The body uses vitamins partly as a means to ensure a healthy immune system; that is to say, to resist disease. The more poisonous our environment is, the more vulnerable we are to infections and other non-infectious diseases, simply because the vitamins in our body are used to protect us. In the West the earth, the air, and food, are all contaminated. We cannot tell exactly what effect defoliants sprayed on the soil, carbon monoxide from cigarettes and from exhaust fumes, and hormones injected into the animals we eat, have on our health. We can, though, be sure that these toxic substances, together with the drugs we take and the thousands of chemicals that are legally added to foods, are draining our bodies of vitamins.

None of this takes dieting into account. What happens when people who are normally getting about half the nourishment their bodies need, go on a diet regime supplying, say, 1000 calories a day? Unless the diet eliminates all sugar, all other processed food, and all food eaten is fresh, lightly cooked and nourishing, their bodies will suffer a sharp shock and will be jerked from a state of mild malnutrition to one of acute, even severe malnutrition.

From the body's point of view, the significant change is not the drop of energy intake; we have always been able to adjust to scarcity and famine, by means which frustrate the dieter. The starvation that the weight-conscious dieter, man or woman, suffers is not of energy but of nourishment.

Here is another reason for the raging appetite dieters develop after the diet has ended. This compulsion for food can so baffle and overwhelm dieters that it becomes a genuinely frightening experience. The healthy body can adjust to a period of emergency, which in effect is what a diet is; but, once the emergency is over, the body's imperative demand is for the nourishment that succours it.

We in the West become overweight against our will, and without being greedy consume more energy from food than our bodies require, because this is the only way our bodies can get enough nourishment. We become overweight as a means of staying healthy. Overweight people who are well known for always being in a good mood are people who have come to terms with being overweight – or, frankly, fat. Their well-being springs not from being overweight, but from getting enough nourishment from food. Such people tend to level out at a weight and percentage of fat well above the 'desirable' level, once the size of their bodies corresponds to a volume of food containing adequate nourishment.

When sedentary or even moderately active people eat sugar and other processed foods the only way they can get enough nourishment is to consume more energy than their bodies require. A vigorously active person can burn off these extra, empty calories; a less active person cannot. Sedentary people have the choice of eventually becoming overweight and then fat; or of being under-nourished and suffering from malaise and then illness. This is why dieters find slimming such a frustrating process. The body's defence and protection mechanisms overpower the mind's desire for the body to become an 'ideal' weight or shape. Ironically, though, in time becoming fat itself is liable to bring illness with it.

> Sugar is an unnecessary source of energy in a community with such a widespread problem of overweight

stated the Royal College of Physicians in their 1983 report on obesity. The report went on to confirm that sugar is not only without value but also deprives us of the vitamins and minerals we would eat in healthy food displaced by sugar:

> A halving of the average sugar consumption per head of the population would increase the nutrient/energy density of the diet. This would ensure that mineral and vitamin requirements were more likely to be met.

Why a halving? Members of the Royal College working party have confirmed to me that their report recommended a halving of processed sugar consumption, rather than cutting it out altogether, for practical, not medical, reasons. The Royal College sees its responsibility to include producing reports that are acceptable not only to the public and to doctors, but also to the Department of Health (DHSS) who will not welcome reports hostile to the interests of the food industry. There is a limit beyond which no representative body is likely to go, in making radical proposals. Nevertheless, the Royal College, in line with reports produced by panels of doctors in America, many European countries and Australia, has made it clear that we have no need of processed sugar and that it deprives us of vitamins and minerals we do need.

Deficiency states

What are the consequences of eating processed sugar? Deficiency diseases are caused by lack of nutrients; by malnutrition, usually, not merely under-nutrition. Some diseases caused by lack of vitamins became epidemic in Western countries in the past among groups in society whose food was very unbalanced, often because of unnatural living conditions, as among the newly industrialised poor, or on board ship. Other such diseases are assumed to be exotic.

Scurvy (caused by lack of vitamin C, also known as ascorbic acid) was commonplace among British sailors, often causing more deaths than battle or shipwreck, until lemons and limes were found to prevent it. Scurvy remained fairly common among poor people who ate no vegetables in winter-time; and rickets (caused by lack of vitamin D) was a common disease among the children of the urban poor in Britain until fifty years ago. Xerophthalmia (lack of vitamin A, or carotene) causes blindness in many children in the Third World, especially Africa. Beri-beri (lack of thiamine, or vitamin B_1) still occurs particularly among people in Asia whose staple cereal is processed white rice. Pellagra (lack of niacin, nicotinic acid, or vitamin B_3) was rampant in the southern states of America among people whose staple diet was corn.

These are the 'classic' deficiency diseases, caused by lack of vitamins whose existence has been known or guessed at for a long time. More vitamins are being identified all the time. The B vitamins are grouped together partly because they tend to work with each other while also having particular vital purposes: other B vitamins include riboflavin (B_2), pyridoxine (B_6), folic acid (also known as folate), cobalamin (B_{12}), and pantothenic acid. All these vitamins have corresponding deficiency states and diseases, which have been identified notably among people who eat mostly processed food.

If we ate whole, nutritious food, and if we were active enough to eat plenty of good food without gaining fat, then we would have less need to be aware of vitamins. Casimir Funk first identified beri-beri as a deficiency disease: it was rampant in the Dutch East Indies at the end of the nineteenth century, not among the very poor, who continued to eat cheap, whole brown rice, but among those who could afford the new polished white rice processed by machines newly imported from Europe. Funk, who coined the term 'vitamin' (meaning 'VITal AMINe') later in his life became an opponent of the commercial system whereby food manufacturers take nutrients out of whole food, defending the practice by adding synthetic versions of some of these nutrients. (Most of the nutrients in white bread, for example, are synthetic. See the table on page 144 in the next chapter, 'Swallow It Whole'). Funk said:

> Vitamins are not any magical possessions. They exist in milk because the mother or the cow assemble them from the food she has eaten. What would be the use of preparing all our foods artificially as long as nature is producing her own foods in sufficient abundance?

Half a century later the USA and the West still produce food in abundance. In November 1982 the total amount of butter, cheese and skimmed milk cached in America was 2399 million pounds; but this dairy produce will not be sold anywhere unless the price is right for the American farmer. Agriculture and food manufacture are very big multinational business. So is the manufacture of vitamin pills.

In their clinical form, caused by gross malnutrition,

deficiency diseases are easy to diagnose. But deficiency states also take mild forms that are not readily identifiable. Dr Donald McLaren, in his standard textbook *Nutrition and Its Disorders*, says:

> Malnutrition means disordered nutrition. Nutrition becomes disordered as a result of any deviation from normal. While gross deviations give rise to frank clinical signs and symptoms and definite biochemical abnormalities it is virtually impossible to draw a line between 'normal' and 'abnormal'.

In common with a growing number of doctors and scientists who have made a special study of the subject, McLaren states that large numbers of people in Western countries are short of vitamins and minerals. Surveys have shown, for example, that thirty-six per cent of American women and twenty-six per cent of Swiss women are short of pyridoxine (vitamin B_6). One reason for this, is that the contraceptive Pill leaches B_6 from the body. Some doctors say that spina bifida is caused by lack of folic acid, B_6, B_{12} and zinc supplied to the baby in the womb.

McLaren himself believes that deficiency of folic acid is particularly common in the West. A nutritionist at the University of Surrey has told me that sixty per cent of a group of people she examined were short of folic acid, and thirty to forty per cent were short of B_6. And she was studying young athletes who ate a lot of food – much of it, though, junk food. American surveys have shown that around a quarter of the population is short of zinc, calcium and magnesium.

What does 'being short of' a vitamin or mineral mean? Panels of doctors and scientists assembled at the request of governments have, all over the world, made recommendations about the amount of vitamins and minerals people need. These are usually known as RDAs ('recommended dietary amounts'). In Britain, RDAs are calculated from the amount needed to avoid manifest clinical deficiency disease, with an arbitrary extra amount added on 'for safety'. For example, in Britain the RDA for vitamin C is thirty mg a day, on the basis that ten mg a day prevents scurvy, and twenty mg is to be on the safe side. In the USA the RDA for vitamin C is sixty mg a day; in the USSR it is seventy-five mg a day. The British government has not got round to asking doctors and scientists to recommend RDAs for most of the vitamins and minerals known since the last War to be vital to health and also to be lacking in processed food.

The British Department of Health states that all but very small sub-sections of the British population are well-fed and get enough vitamins and minerals with their food; and that no accepted survey has shown otherwise. It seems, though, that the only 'accepted' surveys are those commissioned by the Department of Health. No such survey of the British population has been commissioned in recent years. Meanwhile, 'non-accepted' surveys continue to show that a very large percentage of the British population are short of vitamins or minerals.

Professor Michael Crawford, who is responsible for the welfare of the animals at the London Zoo, has pointed out to me that in most cases the recommended dietary amounts of vitamins and minerals specified for farm animals is, weight for weight, higher – sometimes much higher – than for people. Likewise, at the Zoo. It is literally the case that what the Department of Health says will do for people, is reckoned to be inadequate for pigs, cows, monkeys or elephants. I asked Professor Crawford for an explanation. 'At the Zoo' he said 'we are concerned with optimum nutrition'. And farmers cannot afford to husband unhealthy animals.

Doctors, scientists and nutritionists in Britain who are alarmed about this situation, have found it difficult to get the attention of administrators in the Department of Health. Dr John Rivers of the London School of Hygiene and Tropical Medicine has expressed his concern in the scientist's magazine, *Nature*:

> At present where nutrition policies exist at all, they have been evolved by senior administrators in closed cabal with leaders of the health professions. Such cabals will not survive for long . . . It seems likely that general public concern about the role of nutrition in disease, will soon be matched by public demands to be involved in framing the policies necessary for change.

Dr Rivers has been proved wrong. He made his statement in 1979. In the five years that have passed, nothing has changed.

Books are written about individual vitamins. Take one, folic acid. If it is deficient, red blood cells become large, abnormally shaped and short-lived. The result is a form of anaemia, common among women, especially if they need extra nourishment, when menstruating or pregnant. The symptoms are not obvious or sudden and are not likely to be diagnosed as vitamin deficiency. The victim eventually becomes weak, tired, irritable, and sometimes forgetful and sleepy.

And the result? The woman short of folic acid wonders if she could do with a drug, a pep pill or even a bar of chocolate. It is revealing to watch television commercials put out in the afternoon, for mothers and housewives: between the advice shows and the cartoon shows, advertisements for confectionery alternate with advertisements for over-the-counter drugs. The advertisers know what they are doing.

Malnutrition in the West

Doctors acknowledge that a high percentage of their patients complain of unspecific ailments. These include stomach discomfort, loss of appetite, anxiety, backache, constant tiredness, muscle weakness, jumpiness, digestive trouble, headaches, inability to sleep, difficulty in paying attention, nervousness – or 'general malaise', as millions of doctors' certificates put it. Any of these conditions is depressing; all zest for life and sense of well-being is lost. All these complaints can be a result of malnutrition. Certainly, most people in the West do not eat enough nutritious food, and some large groups of people, including students, office workers, old people and dieters, are especially at risk.

Scurvy is generally assumed to have vanished before the end of the sailing ship era. Not at all. In its mild form, scurvy leads to bleeding, notably from the gums, and to fragile bones. Later the joints and muscles bleed, and teeth fall out. McLaren:

> Elderly bachelors and widowers who cook for themselves or eat in restaurants are particularly prone. Women, even when living alone, are better able to fend for themselves, and fruit and vegetables have a more prominent place in their diet.

Vitamin C is used by the body to resist attacks from poisonous substances, such as lead, cadmium, and carbon monoxide from exhaust fumes and from tobacco smoke. Smoking is estimated to lower the vitamin C content of the blood by twenty-five to fifty per cent. Alcohol has a similar effect. So have some drugs—aspirin, for example. The more we are exposed to drugs, poisons and contamination in the air and in our food, the more we need vitamins.

Moreover, foods lose nourishment by being grown in poor soil; by being picked before they are ripe; and by being preserved, dyed or waxed. And no scientist can say what effect the cocktails of chemicals we all eat and breathe is having on our health.

Faced with these facts, confusion and despair tends to set in. What can we do? Short of becoming a campaigner or a crank, an organic farmer or a fugitive from Western culture living on a Greek island, what we can do, today, is to stop eating the one substance that does us no good and can only do us harm: processed sugar.

We need to eat a small amount of salt, and we need to eat fat, too. We eat too much of both salt and fat, and good health depends on eating less of both. With sugar, though, the sensible recommendation is very simple. Cut it out.

Think twice about sugar

Sugar causes deficiency states, especially in sedentary people, because it replaces nourishing food, and because it is a parasitical agent, draining nourishment from the body.

Take beri-beri and pellagra. Vitamin B_1 and vitamin B_3 are lost in cooking, and are attacked by alcohol. They are also both attacked by sugar. Alcoholics in Britain and in other Western countries have been diagnosed as suffering from early stages of beri-beri and pellagra. Beri-beri, or polyneuritis, causes tingling in the hands and feet, mental confusion, and, eventually, heart failure. In mild forms it causes fatigue, weight loss and loss of appetite, exhaustion and sleeplessness, bad memory and mood-

71

swings. Mild pellagra, which is in some respects like mild beri-beri, has been confused with schizophrenia. Every vitamin has a corresponding deficiency disease; every deficiency disease has mild forms often not obvious to doctors, often made worse by drugs.

It may very well be that mild forms of deficiency diseases (also known as 'sub-clinical deficiency diseases' or 'deficiency states') are so common in the West that both the sufferers and their doctors fail to see what the problem is. If I feel ill but nobody else does, I know I have a problem. But if a lot of people feel fairly ill all the time, everybody starts to assume that the condition is normal. How often have you heard somebody who is obviously fit, well and happy described – wrily or enviously – as 'disgustingly healthy'?

It's not all in the mind

It follows that young people, who consume a great deal of convenience and 'junk' food with a high processed sugar content, are especially at risk. So it proves. Dr Derrick Lonsdale and Dr Raymond Shamberger of Cleveland, Ohio, noted symptoms of vitamin B_1 deficiency so severe, among a group of youngsters, as to be recognisable as early forms of beri-beri. Their report, in the *American Journal of Clinical Nutrition*, emphasised their conclusion that their patients were ill from the effects of eating 'empty' or 'naked' calories – energy without nourishment.

The doctors noted severe restlessness during sleep, frightening dreams, and recurrent fever diagnosed as infections by the family doctor. One syndrome was:

> The patient was described as unusually irritable, sensitive to criticism, becoming angered easily and showing poor impulse control, as in the case of a seventeen-year-old male who had put his fist through a plate glass window.

Lonsdale and Shamberger even translated a Japanese treatise on beri-beri into English, finding that many aspects of the disease, 'forgotten in societies where it is believed that the condition is extinct', imitate other well-recognised diseases, because beri-beri affects all the organs and deranges energy metabolism.

How then is it possible to know whether a patient has vitamin B_1 deficiency, rather than some other ailment? The answer is of course in the treatment. The youngsters were given vitamin B_1 supplements – and all of them improved.

Some patients lost their craving for sweet tasting foods and beverages, although in some cases the process was extremely difficult and the temptation to succumb quite similar to that seen in people who express a wish to stop smoking.

The common assumption that diseases of malnutrition only occur among poor people eating simple food is wrong. Just as beri-beri in the East was and is caused by eating white rice, rather than the cheaper brown rice, and little other nutritious food, so Lonsdale and Shamberger's patients were all-American kids eating all-American food.

Many of them had no breakfast at all; most had school lunch and an evening meal was provided at home. In most cases it was between-meals snacking of so-called junk foods, and above all the consumption of a variety of sweet beverages that provided the empty calories.

Almost as an aside, the doctors then make a fascinating deduction from experiments with animals: 'Anorexia may be regarded as a protective device and this is well seen in experimental work with animals who stop eating early in the experiment.'

The suggestion is that young people who eat very little, but who do consume snacks, soft drinks and confectionery as a large part of their diet, are liable to develop a pathological lack of appetite as the body struggles to avoid vitamin B deficiency states. This applies mainly to young women. Young men rarely eat very little and tend to drink alcoholic drinks, such as beer, that supply as well as leach nutrients. Here, then, is a biochemical account of anorexia which suggests that sometimes anorexia nervosa is accurately labelled the 'slimmer's disease'. The body seeks to avoid illness not by

73

consuming too much energy but by rejecting the toxic food altogether. Lonsdale and Shamberger conclude that the consumption of large quantities of soft drinks is a danger to health not yet identified in the USA and other Western countries, and that eating and drinking a lot of junk food can cause intensely disturbing changes in personality and behaviour which parents, teachers and doctors at the moment label as 'the personality of the growing child or adolescent'.

Hyperactive children can be a great trial to their parents and their teachers. Sometimes such children are diagnosed not only as being disturbed – which, indeed, they are – but also as in need of complex, expensive psychoanalytical treatment. With luck and resourceful parents, a hyperactive child may calm down in time. Others may behave in ways that get them classified as delinquent and then, with the passage of time, as criminal.

In common with such children, most of the people who spend periods of their lives in prison, eat bad food. They are likely to have broken homes – and may have come from a broken home. They will find it very difficult to get regular work. They are unlikely to have learned the skills of cooking. It is likely that the food they eat in prison is more nutritious than the food they choose for themselves. A growing number of doctors and nutritionists, especially in America, are now convinced that certain types of criminal behaviour, especially of a bizarre and unpredictable nature, are caused by junk food, and processed sugar in particular. The argument is that the bad food makes these vulnerable people feel bad; and they then act their feelings out.

It sounds an unlikely theory. But, as with the Cleveland study, there is a way to test the theory: give these people good food. Recently in Washington State, California and Virginia, adolescent and adult prisoners were given diets composed of whole food. Their behaviour was monitored as, over periods of weeks or months, they were weaned off white flour, coffee, salted foods, and – in particular – sugar. Violence, aggression and other misbehaviour decreased, in some cases dramatically. This work has also been done in Britain by the Rev Vic Ramsey who, between 1977 – 80, treated around fifty long-stay drug addicts.

Initially with great scepticism, Ramsey and his wife took the patients off convenience foods such as beefburgers, and other foods saturated with salt and sugar, and gave them lightly cooked, fresh whole food. Ramsey said:

> There were colossal changes in behaviour patterns when we gave them good food. They were less aggressive verbally, less violent, less refractory.

I asked John McCarthy for his views. McCarthy is ex-governor of Wormwood Scrubs prison in London, and now director of the Richmond Fellowship, designed to help mental welfare and rehabilitation of prisoners. He said:

> If you are under severe stress, one of the best ways to deal with it is to eat healthy foods. I don't need to be convinced of the psychological changes that can be induced by eating healthy foods. I've seen it all the time.

The junk food syndrome

Students and young office workers are also at risk from deficiency states. Growing boys and girls need significantly more energy from foods than do adults, both to fuel their bodies' growth and for exercise, games and sport. Adolescents who are not especially active nonetheless need about 300 more calories of energy from food than they will five years later. A growing mid-teenage boy who plays a lot of football, say, or other sports will be in energy balance at a level of perhaps 4000 calories a day. A girl of the same age who dances at discos three nights a week will require maybe 3000 calories a day.

Many teenagers who consume a lot of junk food are in danger of deficiency states. But usually they are comparatively healthy; they eat nutritious food as well, and do not have enough money, and maybe not the inclination, to smoke or drink a lot, or consume a great deal of junk food. And there is the pressure of the law and parents' disapproval.

At the age of seventeen or eighteen, all this is liable to

change – dramatically. When the body stops growing, and if, when they become students or start work, young people stop taking exercise, they will require perhaps 1000 calories a day less from food. And most of the energy they do need is for the body's basic functions. The only way to be sure of staying healthy when changing, sometimes literally from one month to the next, from a growing active person to an adult sedentary person, is to eat nothing but nutritious food.

And, typically, this is exactly what students and young office workers do not do. No longer obliged to play games, often living away from home for the first time, with parental influence replaced (certainly in the case of students) by often rather ramshackle ways of life, in a milieu where far more drinking and smoking goes on, and with little money, young adults turn to the food that is cheapest and most available.

Students, especially, resist eating institutional food, but rarely have adequate cooking facilities of their own. So there is a sharp rise in the consumption of very energy-heavy foods with high sugar and fat content: chocolate, biscuits, crisps, peanuts with salt, fried food including chips, soft drinks and colas, takeaways, and beer.

A sedentary person cannot burn off the empty energy in these foods, as an active person can. Sedentary adults, accustomed to eating sugar, are liable to suffer from being badly nourished, and if they then diet will be in a state of acute malnutrition. But the student or young office worker, whose body is unaccustomed to low energy intakes, and who often eats two or even three times the average amount of junk food, is liable to be in an even worse state. And if such young people then go on a diet, they will be in danger of acute illness, which may take a mental or physical form.

My son Ben, when at university, made a habit of cooking fresh food and even of clearing up after himself. He was regarded with a mixture of awe, puzzlement and derision by the other students and was known by them as 'mother'. I asked him to list the malaises and ailments of his fellow students. These included what is often known as the students' syndrome: depression, confusion, torpor, inability to concentrate, sleeplessness, mood swings, aches and pains, colds, discomfort in the gut, pre-menstrual tension, pallor, sweatiness, and an overriding sense that nothing matters. Sophisticates call all this 'existential angst'. Usually it is not caused by failed love affairs, bad marks or the bomb, but by junk food and processed sugar in particular.

And – the other side of the coin – the junk food syndrome is caused by lack of fresh food. Take another vitamin, A (carotene). It is found in green and yellow fruit and vegetables, and in liver. It concentrates in the eyes (which is why lack of it causes blindness in extreme situations) and also in the bloodstream and liver. It is attacked by chemical fertilisers present in foods and by air pollution. Symptoms of vitamin A deficiency include bad skin, sensitive eyes, loss of sense of smell, and inability of the nasal membranes to deal with foreign bodies and germs, leading to hay fever and colds.

When I was at university I did not suffer from malaise and ailments. I ate enough nutritive food on top of sugar-heavy foods and gained two and a half stone in three years. I stayed healthy by getting fat. Young women at college or in their first jobs often go the other way, staying thin while eating more sugar and so becoming ill for lack of nourishment. Ben took another route: he grew in health at university by eating well and being very active physically.

Mothers concerned for the well-being of their children leaving home would do well to ensure that their sons as well as their daughters know what is good food and how to cook good food. Well-nourished students are far less likely to get depressed.

The most popular food sold in Britain is saturated with sugar. Market research shows that four of the twenty top-selling lines in 1981 were 'all chocolate confectionery', 'chocolate biscuits', 'chocolate filled blocks', and 'sweet biscuits'. Also in the same list were 'potato crisps', 'snack products' (some of which are loaded with fat, some with sugar), 'drinks, carbonated, still, cola'; 'drinks, squashes, cordials' and 'drinks, fruit'.

The energy content of 100 grams of potato is about eighty calories; of an apple, about forty calories. Many of the most popular foods, however, are heavy with energy

– not only fats and flour but also chocolate and sweet biscuits, crisps and sweets. All these are more than five times as dense in energy than potatoes, more than ten times as dense in energy than apples. Cornflakes almost reach this level; other popular cereals, such as Sugar Puffs, containing over fifty-six per cent sugar, have a far denser energy content. Flavoured and fruit yoghurts, which have something of a 'health' image, have a sugar content of eighteen per cent – rather more than digestive biscuits.

It sounds sensational to say that millions of people in the West are suffering from mild forms of deficiency diseases, especially when the names of some of the better-known diseases are mentioned – beri-beri, pellagra, scurvy. We think that malnutrition is not a problem in the West partly because we associate malnutrition with starvation. But 'malnutrition' does not mean 'starvation': it means what it says, a state of bad nourishment. And the fact is, that most people in the West are badly nourished. Moreover, we don't think of dieting as starvation, because starvation is not done on purpose, whereas dieting is. But from the body's point of view there's no difference.

Somewhat like baldness and obesity, to some extent it's a matter of judgment whether or not somebody is suffering from the bad food they eat. Unlike drugs, though, good food has no side-effects. No one who feels bad will ever come to any harm from nourishing food.

Children, teenagers, students, young office workers, pregnant women, and old people, are all vulnerable groups of the population, liable to suffer from the effects of eating bad food. So are dieters. For dieters are not only liable to be in a state of malnutrition but also, when on the diet, in a state of semi-starvation.

A rule of thumb for anybody who wants to eat healthy food is: if it's advertised, be careful; if it's canned or packaged, read the label; and if it's got processed sugar in it, don't eat it.

Eating processed food, and sugar in particular, is, then, liable to make us fat, or suffer the effects of malnutrition or – for the unfortunate dieter, yo-yoing from one regime to another, and becoming steadily flabbier – both. That, however, is far from the end of the story.

'Western' diseases

The two vital cores of our bodies and of our health are the alimentary tract, of the stomach and gut; and the cardiovascular system, of the heart, lungs and blood vessels. One is the means to process food, and the other the means to process oxygen – our two fuels.

In the Third World very many people still suffer and die from the infectious diseases that have largely been conquered in the West by improved sanitation and antibiotics. We in the West suffer and die mostly from the so-called 'degenerative' diseases, principally of the alimentary tract and the cardiovascular system. Some of these diseases – constipation, piles, varicose veins, obstructions and irritations of the gut, hernias, ulcers, gallstones, and diabetes, for example – are inconvenient and can be crippling, but are not usually in themselves fatal. Others – heart disease and cancers – are often deadly. Heart disease is now the biggest killer in Great Britain, the USA and other Western countries.

These diseases are rare, sometimes to the point of being practically unknown, in Third World countries not yet touched by Western influence. They are now known as 'Western diseases' or (ironically) the 'diseases of civilisation' because they spread wherever Western influence spreads. When Africans come into the towns from the countryside, when Japanese move to Hawaii, when people from the Yemen move to Israel, when Eskimos give up their traditional way of life, when native Americans on reservations accept white life styles, when people in faraway places have an international airport built in the vicinity, then they always begin to suffer and die from the same diseases as Westerners.

Until recently these diseases were generally known as degenerative diseases, because it was believed that they were a consequence of ageing, and that people in the Third World were free of them simply because life outside the Western world was short. A similar argument has sometimes been mounted to explain why so many people in the West get fat whereas people in the Third World living traditional lives as a rule do not; the

79

argument was that Third World people just didn't live long enough.

It is of course true that, in general, life expectancy in Western countries is higher than in the Third World. But life expectancy at the age of forty is much the same in many non-Western countries as it is in the West; and all countries and societies contain plenty of people who live the Biblical three score years and ten, and longer still. Moreover, many such people have eaten well, and have not lived very active lives, typically going out to fish or hunt or work in the fields about as often as pre-machine age people did in Western countries. And the fact is that old people in the Third World, living in the country, do not as a rule suffer or die from the so-called 'degenerative' diseases. What then is the cause of these diseases, the scourge of Western societies?

It is now generally agreed, by doctors who study the incidence of disease in different societies and different countries, that the main cause of the diseases most of us in the West suffer and die from is the food we eat. Above everybody else, the doctor who proposed the causal connection between Western food and Western disease with most force was Surgeon-Captain T L (Peter) Cleave, who during his professional life as a Royal Navy officer, studied patterns of disease and nutrition notably by means of voluminous correspondence with doctors and scientists all over the world.

Food: the key to health

Western doctors are still taught to regard food as incidental to health. If nutrition had its proper, central place in Western medicine, Cleave would have received a Nobel Prize; as it is, he did more than any other individual to remind doctors and lay people alike of the vital role of food in health. Much of the power of his argument lies in its essential simplicity.

In 1956 he published a long paper in the *Journal of the Royal Naval Medical Service*: 'The Neglect of Natural Principles in Current Medical Practice'. A keen natural historian in the tradition of Darwin, he wrote:

No rabbit ever ate too much grass, no rook ever pulled up too many worms, no herring ever caught too much plankton: no creature in the wild state is ever over-weight. They may vary in size, but never in shape.

He proposed that the key difference between the food we eat and the food animals eat is that much of our food is processed; that is to say, concentrated by machinery developed as means of mass manufacture only in the last 100 or 150 years. For Cleave the villain of all the foods we eat is processed sugar and starch:

> Wholemeal flour is turned into white flour, and the bran rejected; the pulp of the sugar cane and the sugar beet have the sugar extracted in almost pure form, and the balance of the pulp is then likewise rejected. Now whereas cooking has been going on in the human race for probably 200,000 years . . . there is no question yet of our being adapted to the concentration of carbohydrates by machinery. Such procedures have been in existence for little more than a century for the common man.

Cleave went on to write short books on heart disease, stomach ulcers and diabetes in which he traced the rise of these and other Western diseases, showing the link between them and the rise of consumption of Western foods, processed sugar in particular. He also proposed bodily mechanisms by which Western food causes diseases. His last book, *The Saccharine Disease*, was published in 1974, and has had a profound impact on leading doctors in the West. Sir Richard Doll, Emeritus Professor of Medicine at Oxford University, and the man who jointly established the connection between smoking and lung cancer, has repeatedly stated recently that perhaps thirty per cent of all cancers are caused by the food we in the West eat. In a preface to one of Cleave's books Sir Richard wrote that if only a small amount of Cleave's thinking proved to be true he 'will have made a bigger contribution to medicine than most university departments or medical research units make in the course of a generation.'

Sir Francis Avery Jones, a distinguished doctor who specialises in diseases of the gut, has gone further, saying

81

that the work of Cleave and his supporters 'will prove to be, after antibiotics, the most important medical advance of this century'.

Western diseases are not 'inherited'

The title of Cleave's book, *The Saccharine Disease*, reflects his thesis that many Western diseases are properly seen as various manifestations of a single master disease, caused by eating processed, concentrated sugar and starch, which both convert into sugar in the body. Cleave has always dismissed the idea, commonly stated by doctors, that Western diseases are 'inherited'. If so, he points out, why is it that such diseases are practically confined to people living Western-style lives, and are rare or unknown in the wild? Diseases of proven genetic origin are rare; necessarily so, states Cleave, because living creatures are all evolved in harmony with their environment. Any species in which hereditary defects were common would have become extinct. The fault is not in ourselves, nor in nature, but in our modern man-made life-style.

It is true that disease can be transmitted from the mother to the child growing in the womb. Countless animal experiments have shown that the off-spring of badly fed females are liable to be born defective or else to develop disease after birth, and to live short lives. The official government view in Britain is that generally speaking our food is so good that only tiny sections of the population get inadequate nourishment from their food. In 1982 Professor Michael Crawford and Wendy Doyle of the Nuffield Institute of Human Nutrition in Regent's Park made two studies of pregnant women in London; one in the working-class area of Hackney, the other in the middle-class district of Hampstead. They found that even judged by the official 'minimum plus' standards, the food of most of the Hackney mothers was short of many vitamins and minerals. As a consequence, their babies were being born light in weight; in some cases, so much so as to be medically at risk. Low birth-weight is associated with various physical and mental defects. There was no such problem with the Hampstead babies. Much of the food the Hampstead mothers ate was fresh. Almost all of the food the Hackney mothers ate, was processed sugar and starch and other food soaked in fat.

But to say that a disease can be transmitted from mother to child is not to say that its cause is heredity. Even when a disease is transmitted from generation to generation the cause may nevertheless be something in the environment.

We are all born with constitutions that are more, or less, strong, and with different parts of the body that are more, or less, resilient. People who doubt the causal connection between smoking and lung cancer, sometimes refer to the fabulous eighty-year-old man who is hale and hearty on sixty cigarettes a day. If any such man has thrived (and I'm sceptical; he always seems to be someone else's grandfather) he merely proves that some people are born with exceptionally resilient lungs.

What Cleave proposes, is that processed and concentrated sugars and starches, and above all processed sugar, are the agent, which is to say the cause, of various Western diseases. Which of these diseases we eventually suffer and die from will largely depend on our constitutional make-up. Some people will develop stomach ulcers, diverticular disease, cancer of the bowel, or other conditions to which they are predisposed by action of bad food on a sensitive gut. Other people will develop diabetes, heart disease or strokes, or other conditions indicating that they have a system of blood supply liable to be deranged by bad food. Everybody will develop tooth decay; and very many people will become overweight or obese. And, of course, some people will develop clusters of these diseases and disabilities, all of which, Cleave states, are liable to have the same fundamental cause, and all of which rarely occur in people who do not eat Western-influenced food.

Sugar and the gut

Many Western ailments and diseases are of the alimentary tract or gut. Almost everybody in the West is constipated to some extent. It is well known that constipation is caused by a lack of fibre (previously commonly known as 'bulk' or 'roughage') in the food we eat. The condition is eased by eating bran as a supplement to food. The basic cause of constipation, though, is that the sugars and starches we eat are typically stripped of the fibre to be found in whole food.

Constipation, hiatus hernia, varicose veins and piles, are rare in rural communities in the Third World. Cleave, and a body of doctors with clinical experience especially in Africa, state that the large quantities of whole starchy food eaten in the Third World allows food to pass more rapidly through the alimentary tract, giving the gut work it is designed to do, and leading to the formation of large soft stools.

By contrast, the constant straining caused by the bullet-like material formed from processed and concentrated starch and sugar, is a direct cause of hernia, varicose veins and piles. Cleave goes further, and proposes that the constant irritation, friction and pressure of constipation is a prime cause of more serious conditions, such as diverticular disease (a kind of rupture of the colon, common among middle-aged people in the West). Moreover, there is evidence that cancers of the large bowel and colon are caused by the stagnant stools of Western people, containing toxins that cannot be neutralised by the bacteria in the gut. Cleave states:

> The frequency of cancer increases steadily in each successive part of the colon, cancer of the rectum being one of the commonest in the body. It is significant that the irritant effect of any toxins on the intestinal wall must increase steadily in each of these successive parts, both on account of the actual greater production of toxins, and also on account of the progressive slowing that normally occurs in the colonic contents as they pass onwards.

In the nineteenth century it became understood that the irritants in soot caused skin cancer in chimney sweeps. In the last thirty years, it has become accepted that the irritants in cigarette smoke cause cancers of the mouth, tongue, throat, bronchial passages and lungs of smokers as well as conditions such as bronchitis not in themselves normally deadly. The proposal that processed sugar is a major cause of cancers of the lower gut has a similar basis; that the hard, toxic and offensive stools formed from sugar and other processed foods, are a constant irritant to the gut, day after day, year after year.

The cause, or agent, of tooth decay, is of course processed sugar. Almost all the qualified people who dispute this fact are either employees of the sugar industry or else funded by the sugar or food industries. Half a century ago the American dentist Weston Price spent nine years of his later life travelling the world, documenting the condition of the teeth of many communities, for his book *Nutrition and Physical Degeneration*. In this epic work, he invariably found that when people ate traditional whole food, their teeth remained sound throughout life. He reinforced his point by examining the teeth of thousands of skeletons. He also found that when people started to eat Western food their teeth became rotten. Worse yet, as the title of his book indicates, he found that when parents switched from whole to processed food, their elder children were born with well-formed jaws, but their young children's teeth frequently grew crushed together in a malformed jawline. When parents eat processed food, their children suffer.

Sugar and heart disease

Sugar has a directly harmful effect on the alimentary tract. Does it also harm the cardiovascular system? The food we eat in the West is bad for our health not only because it is heavy in sugar and in processed starch such as white flour and white bread. We also eat far too much animal fat. Animals today are bred to be fat, and so the meat we eat is far fattier than it was in our grandparents' day. Masses of fatty waste from animal carcasses is used to make cheap foods such as sausages and beefburgers. We consume a lot of full-fat dairy products such as milk, butter and cheese. In America and France milk with the fat skimmed off is generally available; not so in Britain.

And we also eat quantities of fat made palatable by the addition of sugar, as chocolate and confectionery.

Heart attacks and strokes are preceded by the build-up of certain types of fat in the blood, which in turn lead to the build-up of fatty deposits on the inside of blood vessels. Thus the blood vessels in the body, heart and brain are narrowed. This process can be compared with the furring of domestic water pipes. High blood pressure ('hypertension') is a warning sign that the blood vessels are becoming silted up with fatty deposits ('atherosclerosis'). Eventually the vessels become so narrow that a blood clot ('thrombus') is liable to form. Should the clot block the blood vessels of the brain the result is a stroke ('cerebral thrombosis'). If the blood vessels of the heart are blocked the result is a heart attack ('coronary thrombosis').

Since half the deaths in Britain today are caused by heart attacks and strokes, we have a powerful reason to find out what causes the build-up of fat in the blood and on the walls of blood vessels.

Heart disease is typically described as 'multifactorial' in origin; meaning, that it has many causes. Doctors are not the only professional people in the habit of making things sound more complicated than they actually are. Take heart disease.

One cause of heart disease is a weak heart, and weak blood vessels. If the muscle of the heart lacks strength, and if the blood vessels covering the heart itself, and throughout the body, degenerate, then we become more vulnerable to heart attacks. And, as a recent campaign of the Health Education Council rightly states, 'action makes the heart grow stronger'. (The next chapter, 'More Air! More Air!' explains why and how exercise of the right type strengthens the heart and regenerates the blood vessels.)

Another cause of heart disease, is bad blood; not of course in the sense that leads to knife fights in Sardinia, but in the sense of blood containing too much of the wrong type of blood fat. In particular, scientists have recently made a vital distinction between 'high density lipoprotein' and 'low-density lipoprotein'. It is now

86

understood that the problem is not fat in the blood; but the type of fat in the blood. 'High density lipoprotein' (HDL), which is fat (lipid) bound up with protein, consists of tiny globules, smooth to the point of being abrasive; one of its functions may be to scour the inside surfaces of blood vessels, as a sort of natural Vim. 'Low-density lipoprotein', by contrast, consists of relatively large globules, and is sticky. Healthy blood has a high proportion of HDL. Unhealthy blood has a high proportion of LDL. LDL is behind the build-up of cholesterol in the blood, and high cholesterol levels are known to increase the risk of a heart attack. So, what causes a high proportion of LDL?

As soon as it became known that a major cause of heart disease is the build-up of certain types of fat in the blood, dietary fat became the popular villain. Nowadays people are liable to believe that eating fat is a bad idea because, well, fat is fat: without a knowledge of human biochemistry we assume that fat in the blood (or, indeed, body fat) is made from dietary fat – the fat we eat as butter, or in meat, chocolate, sausages or milk. In fact, though, the human body does not merely turn a dietary substance into its equivalent in the body.

Once upon a time athletic coaches thought that the only way to build up their champions was to feed them meat, because, well, meat is animal muscle. So boxers and football stars were fed steaks. In fact, it is just as sensible to feed cereal to athletes; the body converts starch into energy for the muscles, and cereal also contains protein. There again, confectioners sell their goods by associating processed sugar with blood sugar, suggesting that active children need candy bars; whereas, once again, starch is a better source of energy.

In the case of fat, the story is not so simple. It is certain that we in the West eat far too much fat, notably animal fat, as meat, dairy products and in many convenience foods, and it is certain that animal fat, eaten in excess, is a prime cause of the build-up of the wrong kinds of fat in the blood and in turn of fatty deposits on the walls of blood vessels. The next chapter ('Swallow It Whole') recommends that we eat much less fat, especially animal fat.

At the same time, though, anything else we eat that causes bad blood, in the sense of increasing the proportion of LDL in the blood, and increasing the tendency of fat in the blood to deposit itself on the inside walls of blood vessels, will therefore also increase the risk of a heart attack.

T.L. Cleave made a study of the rise of heart disease in the West and showed that, in country after country, that rise was preceded by an acceleration in processed sugar consumption. In Britain for example, the great rise in sugar consumpion, almost to today's levels, occurred towards the end of the nineteenth century, and the great rise in heart disease started about twenty years later. In the early years of this century heart disease was uncommon.

The Rule of Seventy and Twenty

Doctors who study the patterns of health and disease in populations, are known as epidemiologists. (The word comes from the Greek 'epi' meaning 'upon'; 'demos' meaning 'people'; and 'logos' meaning 'study': so literally it means 'the study of what comes upon people'. Hence, 'epidemic'.) In the case of sugar, epidemiologists have proposed 'The Rule of Seventy and Twenty'. This points to the fact that various Western diseases, including heart disease, and also obesity, become epidemic around twenty years after a population starts to eat more than seventy pounds of processed sugar a year.

The 'Rule of Seventy and Twenty' is an effective rule of thumb. Other Western diseases, notably of the stomach and gut, seem to take rather longer to develop. On the other hand, diabetes can develop with startling speed in populations introduced to sugar by a process of 'Coca-colonisation'. Their bodies have a low tolerance for processed sugar.

The 'Rule of Seventy and Twenty' works well as a means to predict the onset of Western diseases, and this is one of its strengths. It was this kind of evidence that first established the causal link between cigarette smoking and

88

lung cancer. But in the case of heart disease, its spread is also preceded by a general increase in the amount of fat eaten – and, notably, fat of low quality. Moreover, fat is known to be an important cause of heart disease.

The clinical evidence

In the 1960s Professor John Yudkin fed high levels of processed sugar to nineteen student volunteers and after some weeks found that:

> dietary sucrose can be shown in experiment to produce several of the disturbances seen in coronary thrombosis

After a period of weeks, Yudkin had found that the blood of some of his volunteers – who were eating around three times as much sugar as they would normally eat – could be shown in a laboratory to have become more sticky, and fattier. He also found that there was more insulin in the blood: this increases the risk of diabetes and also of heart disease. The blood of a majority of the volunteers did not react in this way; the explanation given, being that only a proportion of the population is sensitive to processed sugar, and were it otherwise, we would all develop diabetes and have heart attacks.

Yudkin is a well-known campaigner against processed sugar; he has written a book on the subject called *Pure, White and Deadly*. His experimental results and his views have always been vehemently attacked by the representatives and the supporters of the world sugar trade, who have always been better organised than the defenders of animal fat. It is now commonly assumed that Yudkin's results were suspect – 'untypical', as scientists politely say. Yet in 1983, in his contribution to the book *Medical Applications Of Clinical Nutrition*, Dr Sheldon Reiser reviewed well over a hundred clinical studies most of which supported Yudkin's work. These studies showed that when animals, or human volunteers, were fed high levels of sugar, the level of insulin, and the level of low density lipoprotein, in the blood, increased. Furthermore, when volunteers cut down or completely cut out their consumption of sugar, undesirable types of fat in the blood dropped. These results were found in a proportion of subjects, evidently vulnerable to sugar. Reiser also noted that processed sugar and animal fat seem to work together in combination.

The case against processed sugar is mounting. Meanwhile it is certain that nobody ever came to any harm from cutting it out, totally.

Confusion or cover-up?

Food manufacturers, as well as sugar manufacturers and importers, are as reluctant to accept the dangers of processed sugar, as cigarette manufacturers are to accept that smoking is deadly. Indeed, the problem with sugar is bigger than the problem with tobacco: sugar is mixed into every kind of food.

The defenders of processed sugar have also made much of two potentially muddling points about sugar. First, for many years food scientists made the disastrous mistake of grouping sugar and starch together as 'carbohydrate' (the reason being that both sugar and starch supply energy to the body). Second, it still is not generally understood why processed sugar is bad for us, whereas natural sugar (in fruit and some vegetables) is good for us. What's the difference?

The body needs sugar for all its functions. Body sugar is made from carbohydrates; and starchy foods such as cereals, bread, pasta and certain vegetables are as good a source of sugar for the body as are sweet foods. A proper level of blood sugar is essential for physical and mental well-being, and a sandwich or plate of spaghetti a day does indeed help you work, rest and play.

So do the fruits and vegetables containing natural sugar. 'Sugar in Food', the table accompanying this chapter on pages 102 – 5, lists foods high in natural sugar, which are nutritious. They contain many vitamins, minerals and other nutrients, and also the fibre the body needs, as well as energy for the body from sugar.

Processed sugar poisons the body, not because it is sugar, but because it is processed. Other processed foods such as white flour and white rice are also drained of nourishment and cause illness if eaten to the exclusion of nourishing food. Thus a sedentary person who, as well as eating sugar, also eats white flour in cakes and biscuits makes bad worse. But white flour has some nourishment in it, although far less than wholemeal flour.

One question underlies all other question about sugar. It is simply this. Why, if it is true that processed sugar is a poison, do we eat it?

Professor Yudkin's answer, that sugar is 'highly palatable', obviously has some truth in it. But why should the body accept the amount of sugar we eat, given that processed sugar has such disastrous effects on our health and well-being? The explanation that sugar is 'highly palatable' seems thin. Another answer, suggested by political radicals such as Hannah Wright of the *New Statesman*, that sugar is cheap, does not rot, is easily transported, heavily advertised and very profitable obviously has truth in it. In 1979 British press and television advertising for processed sugar and sugar-heavy products totalled £60 million, and advertising works. But this explanation is rather thin, too; a product must be attractive in the first place, before advertising will work. Sugar has a magnetism unique among all substances we eat and drink. What is it in processed sugar that overwhelms the body's defences?

The answer lies in the nature of the disease which, after tooth decay, is most unequivocally caused by processed sugar: adult onset diabetes.

Diabetes: the sugar disease

Thomas Willis, the seventeenth-century doctor who first identified diabetes after noting the sweet-smelling urine of his rich patients, wrote in 1685, in Latin, 'I do much disapprove things preserved or very much sweetened with sugar'. And he intuitively realised that eating food containing energy but no nourishment can cause vitamin deficiency diseases, saying of sugar, 'I judge the invention of it and its immoderate use to have very much contributed to the vast increase of scurvy in this last age'.

91

Dr Willis waited before publishing his views. He had been court physician to King Charles II, who had enjoyed the revenue from the slave trade and so from processed sugar. It would not have been tactful for Willis to press his point. And from that day to this, many well-placed doctors have minced their words about the relationship between processed foods and disease. Indeed, most doctors and scientists whose views on food are well-publicised, are consultants to the food industry.

Word about the connection between processed sugar and diabetes is now, however, getting out; in large part because the epidemiological evidence is now very strong. In the 1980 report on dietary fibre, the Royal College of Physicians noted:

> A high prevalance of diabetes seems to be characteristic of recently urbanised populations. Examples are Indians and Zulus in South Africa, Yemeni Jews in Israel, American Indians throughout the United States, Maoris in New Zealand, and Polynesians in the Central Pacific island of Nauru. The dietary change which has most often been blamed has been the adoption of refined sugar.

The exploitation of phosphates to be found on Nauru has brought the islanders the highest per capita income in the world; but at the price of their health. Dr Denis Burkitt has told me that the incidence of diabetes on Nauru has been estimated at forty-two per cent. But when Alexander Frater visited the island for the *Observer* in October 1982, a European nurse there told him that the incidence was ninety per cent. Dr Thoma, head of medical services, said to Frater:

> We have the second highest rate of diabetes in the world, after the Pima Indians of Phoenix, Arizona. The disease can be prevented and controlled by diet. People here eat too much, and the food is all canned and refined.

Dr Frederick Banting isolated insulin in the 1920s. He regarded it as a palliative, not a cure, for diabetes. He had little doubt about the cause of diabetes in adults. His own observations told Banting that natural sugar is a food but processed sugar is a poison. In 1924 he visited Panama and spoke to a doctor examining men applying for work on the Panama Canal, who had found evidence of diabetes in the urine of two men only – neither of whom proved to be diabetic. Banting commented:

> This is the more remarkable because a large percentage of the labourers were natives of Dominica, where a main article of diet was sugar-cane. From the time the children are weaned until they die they eat the sugar-cane. There are also wealthy Spaniards who live in Panama who eat large quantities of refined cane sugar. Indeed much of their food is cooked in syrup. The incidence of diabetes amongst this class is surprisingly high.

Foods containing sugar in its natural state – bananas, oranges, apples, grapes and other fruits, sweet potato, onions, carrots and other vegetables, and the cane and beet from which sugar is processed – are nutritious and good for us. The cause of diabetes is not sugar, but sugar in an intensely concentrated form. Diabetes could theoretically develop from eating massive amounts of honey, which is sugar refined by bees, or dried fruits such as dates, raisins, sultanas and currents. But we are satisfied by small amounts of these foods, which are to be avoided only by diabetics. Also, honey and dried fruits are nutritious.

So how is diabetes caused? Our good health and sense of well-being depends on the level of sugar in our blood being neither too high, nor too low. Hunger is triggered when the level of sugar in the blood falls below a certain point. Starches and sugars, when eaten, both raise blood-sugar levels. Starches, eaten in the form of cereals, bread or pasta, or potatoes, say, raises the blood-sugar at a natural speed; as do the sugars in fruit and vegetables which, bound up in the body of the food when eaten, seep into the bloodstream. The sense of fullness and satisfaction derived from eating such foods is reliable, especially when the flour in bread or in the pasta is wholewheat (and therefore not robbed of fibre, vitamins and minerals).

But because of its concentration, processed sugar shoots into the bloodstream and is liable to raise the blood-sugar level too high. The immediate effect of this sugar rush is very pleasant and is used to good effect in advertisements of products saturated with sugar, in which people look happy. But after a certain point, eating sugar becomes nauseating: this is especially noticeable if the initial blood-sugar level is very low, as it is in a runner after a long-distance race or a dieter, both of whom feel the need for sugar but can suffer if they eat a candy bar rather than fruit or a sandwich.

When the level of blood-sugar becomes too high, the body lowers it by releasing insulin from the pancreas into the bloodstream. The faster the blood-sugar level rises, and the higher it goes, the more intense and sudden the reaction of the pancreas. This 'panic' reaction results in too much insulin being poured into the bloodstream, so that, paradoxically, the result of eating or drinking food saturated with processed sugar is to change the blood-sugar level from too high to too low. Medically this phenomenon is known as 'rebound hypoglycaemia'. ('Hypo' means low, as 'hyper' means high; and 'glycaemia' refers to glucose, or 'blood-sugar'.)

The 'asleep at the wheel' syndrome

In due course this over-sensitisation of the pancreas is liable to lead to a condition which can be termed 'hyperinsulinism' or 'hypoglycaemia', a doctors' term for the whiplash effect of eating and drinking refined sugar or alcoholic drinks, which have the same result. Hypoglycaemia has been in vogue recently, partly because Richard Harris and Julie Andrews have both revealed that they are sufferers, because of alcohol and sweets respectively. As Julie Andrews confessed to *Woman* magazine: 'If I made the foolish mistake of having a brownie when I thought I was going to have an easy day and could indulge myself, I had the most awful fatigue and dizziness. You wouldn't believe it.'

This state can be dangerous. The one time I fell asleep at the wheel, was after running a half-marathon on a hot day, after which I ate two 'Marathon' candy bars which the race organisers had supplied to the runners. (This was before I had done the research for this book!) Half-an-hour after the race I was driving home, fast, down a motorway, and without any warning fell unconscious, and was jerked awake only by my head hitting the steering wheel.

The contrast in public knowledge about the relationship between food and health in America and Britain is reflected in the fact that Perrier water is a sponsor of the New York marathon; whereas in 1984 the major sponsor of the London marathon is Mars Bars (who also manufacture the Marathon bar, known in America as a 'Snicker').

Sugar makes you hungry, because sugar in its processed form has the paradoxical effect of lowering blood-sugar levels and setting up a need for the very food that converts artificially quickly into blood-sugar – that is, processed sugar. The dependency thus set up, drives out the natural desire for starchy and sweet whole foods that supply blood-sugar at a natural rate, because that rate comes to feel too slow. The body of someone who eats an average amount of processed sugar is liable to alternate from being too high, to being too low, in blood-sugar. Balance is destroyed. The natural patterns of mood, emotion, sleep, energy and fatigue, concentration and reverie, are invaded and confused.

Sugar is with us all the time. It is a term of endearment. It is a comfort.

> The habit of eating for pleasure or comfort such high energy foods as sweets, chocolates, cakes, biscuits and desserts is initiated in childhood. These items may be given out for good behaviour, and withheld as punishment

points out the Royal College of Physicians' report on obesity; which goes on to suggest, reasonably enough, that, so trained, adults will turn to such foods when anxious or depressed.

Sugar is one of the things 'little girls are made of'. Babies are kept quiet by sweet water rubbed on their dummies. The new-born infant prefers sugar solution to water. An American study found that:

> Compared with infants not fed sweetened water, the infants fed sweetened water ingested more sucrose solution but not

95

more water at six months of age. Those infants not fed sweetened water exhibited a diminished intake of sucrose solution relative to water at six months of age.

That is to say, give sugar to a tiny baby, and it will learn to want more of it. Children so small that they cannot see over the counter beg the assistant for sweets; and chocolates are a conventional gift for a loved one. In service stations, newspaper shops, supermarket checkouts, sweets are the impulse buy. In Britain the last course at table or in a restaurant, the naughty temptation, is called 'the sweet'. On average, everyone in Britain eats a ton of processed sugar every twenty years. How can it be that it is so common, so attractive, and yet so bad for us?

Why sugar makes you fat – and worse

Together with alcohol, processed sugar has a special quality that causes the sugar eater to gain fat. Discussions of energy balance tend to treat it like a bank balance: put too much energy in and you get fat, put less energy in and you get thin. People who defend sugar always make a lot of this idea, pointing out that carbohydrates, including sugar, have an energy value of 3.75 calories per gram, compared with 4.1 calories per gram for protein and the much higher figure of 9.3 calories per gram for fat (the figures are often quoted as 4: 4: 9, but these are more precise). The boldest defenders of processed sugar, such as the British Sugar Bureau, set up to protect the interests of Tate & Lyle and British Sugar, which runs an operation from London's Park Lane headed by Michael Shersby, a Conservative Member of Parliament, go so far as to suggest that sugar is therefore a low-energy food and an essential part of any weight reducing regime!

Even allowing that the body can be seen as a bank, this argument is specious. Foods containing sugar are indeed low-energy foods – when they are whole foods, whose natural sugar is bound up with fibre, and with other nutrients, and water. A pound of apples, for example, has an energy content of around 175 calories; a pound of grapes, 225 – 275 calories. Apples include around twelve per cent natural sugar; grapes, around thirteen to sixteen per cent natural sugar. Four ounces of sweets, by comparison, amount to 300 – 500 calories; sweets are little more than processed sugar, some, like toffee, with added fat. And as well as being nourishing, apples and grapes will be more satisfying than sweets, simply because of their bulk: they are more filling. It is only when sugar occurs naturally in whole foods that it can honestly be described as 'low-energy'.

Processed sugar is not of course the only thing we eat that can make us fat. Since the turn of this century, the amount of dietary fat people in Britain and other Western countries eat, expressed as a percentage of total calories consumed, has increased from thirty per cent to around forty to forty-two per cent. Consequently, we nowadays eat about ninety-five pounds of fat per person per year – almost as much fat as sugar, in terms of quantity, supplying twice as many calories as sugar. One reason is that much of the meat we eat comes from animals bred to be fatty, to conform to European farming regulations. It is prudent to eat less meat, and to eat lean meat – such as poultry without its skin.

Another reason why we eat more fat, is that food manufacturers make fat palatable by adding processed sugar to fat. We have a natural taste for sweet things; our tongues have sensors specifically to appreciate sweetness. This is why children like sweets; but you do not see children eating bars of lard or spoonfuls of butter. Much of the food we eat that is heavy in fat is loaded with sugar – chocolate bars, for example, ice-cream, cakes and biscuits. Eat less sugar, and you are very likely indeed to eat less fat.

But the human body is not just a piggy bank for food. The body reacts to different types of food in different ways. In particular, any food that has the effect of over-stimulating a healthy pancreas will tend to make you fat for reasons which have nothing to do with the energy content of the food. The reason is as follows. The insulin poured into the bloodstream as a result of the pancreas being over-stimulated does not merely 'dissolve' the blood sugar, as some books suggest. The story does not end there. The insulin gets rid of the blood sugar by a process that, first, converts the blood-sugar into low-density lipoprotein, the type of blood-fat that is implicated in heart disease; and then, second, dumps this fat running free in the blood into the store of fatty tissue.

This is why sugar concentrated, by processing, has a fundamentally different effect on the body than sugar naturally occurring in whole foods like fruit. It follows that the higher the concentration of processed sugar in food, the greater the impact on the pancreas. Soft drinks like Coca-Cola are an example, because the water with which the sugar in soft drinks is diluted, does not have a protective effect. Confectionery like chocolate, Mars Bars and Bounty Bars, all of which are more than half processed sugar, mixed with fat, are also liable to over-stimulate the pancreas and so make you doubly fat.

Why children should not eat sweets

Vigorously active people can consume processed sugar and not get fat, for reasons touched on in the last chapter, and enlarged upon in chapter 5 ('More Air! More Air!'). If the muscles or the liver are low in glycogen, then the insulin released by the pancreas will convert blood-sugar into glycogen. Bearing in mind that glycogen in the body is bound up with water, this is why a dieter's 'binge' on sweet things is not only so compulsive but also has such a dramatic effect on body weight.

There again, people who run about a lot, as children naturally do, or who play sport a lot, as schoolchildren ordinarily do, are using the glycogen in their muscles all the time. So a Coca-Cola or a Mars Bar is liable to be converted not into body fat, but muscle glycogen. Only active people can efficiently use processed sugar as body fuel. This does not mean – whatever the soft drink and confectionery manufacturers may tell you – that the body of an active person has any *need* for processed sugar. As already stated, starchy foods convert just as readily into glycogen.

Besides, processed sugar 'hits' abuse the pancreas of active and sedentary people, alike. Mothers who want to ensure that their children do not become diabetic in later life should feed them with plenty of wholewheat bread, with sugar-free spreads. (There is also reason to believe that constant over-stimulation of any gland, of which the pancreas is one, becomes addictive in time, and that people who, when children, consumed a lot of processed sugar, are liable when adult to turn to alcohol, especially spirits, which have the same effect on the pancreas. The child's candy becomes the adult's Gin).

For sedentary people, the hormone insulin reacts to processed sugar in a way which makes them fat. Hypoglycaemia, the pre-diabetic state, is a consequence of an abused pancreas nevertheless still capable of over-reacting to the processed sugar 'rush'. A hypoglycaemic person is particularly liable to gain fat, and therefore particularly likely to try one futile diet regime after another. Sad to say, the weight problem of a hypoglycaemic person is liable to be eased only by the onset of diabetes.

Medical textbooks tend to associate diabetes with obesity. In this, they are misleading. Obesity is, rather, fairly likely to be a signal of a pre-diabetic state. Diabetes in adults is caused by an abused pancreas eventually becoming exhausted, and packing up. Then, the process whereby insulin converts sugar to fat in the blood, and thence to fat in the body, ceases. Instead, the blood sugar is, first, dumped into the kidneys, and then into the urine, and thereafter builds up to dangerous levels which are deadly unless checked.

It follows, therefore, that a rather sudden weight loss, especially in adults in their forties or fifties who had previously been gaining fat on a Western diet, is a signal that a pre-diabetic state has become clinical diabetes.

Professor Harry Keen of Guys Hospital is a leading specialist who is disinclined to agree that sugar is to blame for diabetes. Nevertheless, in 1975 he published a highly significant study. He asked 711 people diagnosed as diabetic to recall their heaviest weight in the past; and also weighed them. He repeated the process with relatives of the diabetics, and with a 'control' group of unrelated non-diabetics. He found that the weight of the diabetics was much the same as that of the other people. The one outstanding finding was that on average, the diabetics had weighed twenty pounds more, before being diagnosed as diabetic. That is to say, these people, pre-diabetic, were on average one and a half stone heavier than they were when clinically diabetic.

People who consume more energy than their bodies need, will gain fat. Processed sugar makes you fat, for three reasons. First, it has no nourishment in it and therefore cheats the body's natural desire for nourishment. Second, it is concentrated and therefore heavy in energy, and therefore deceives the appetite, which is naturally satisfied by whole, bulky foods. Third, and most important, processed sugar makes us fat because it disturbs the hormone, insulin. Processed sugar is the link between obesity, diabetes and heart disease.

Sedentary people who eat an average amount of processed sugar (or who drink a lot of alcohol) face one of two dismal futures. Either they will eat enough nutritious food, and the sugar on top, in which case they will end up overweight or even obese, and be liable to suffer from diabetes, heart disease or other Western diseases in middle age. Or, they will avoid gaining weight in the only way sedentary people can, by eating half or maybe even less of the nourishing food their bodies need, in which case the result will be malaise, debilitation, and eventually chronic deficiency states – the junk food syndrome.

Sugar addiction

But if processed sugar is deadly, why do our bodies accept it? What is the overwhelming attraction of sugar? The answer is in front of our eyes every day, in service stations, newspaper shops, supermarkets and restaurants. Imagine the reaction of a child refused sweets, or of adults told there is no sugar for their tea or coffee. The child will make a fuss; may even filch money to buy sweets, or steal the sweets from the shop. The adults will fidget; may refuse the drink, and be pleased if you borrow a cup of sugar from a neighbour. Such behaviour is so usual and expected that we do not realise how striking and strange it is. The mother distrusts her child, and why? Because the child has stolen pennies from her purse. And what for? To buy sweets.

The Department of Health and Social Security, in an official document published in 1975, had this to say:

> Better dental health could be assured if only parents discouraged children from eating sweets, lollipops, drinks containing sugar and so on . . . but childhood without sweets may well be regarded by many as a fate worse than an adulthood without teeth.

If processed sugar were unknown and were now introduced, and its effects observed, it would be made illegal. We shy away from the word 'addictive', tending to use it only of substances which, as well as being poisonous, are illegal. But, after all, it was only 200 years ago that mothers quietened their babies by means of opium smeared on a little finger. Later, opium became illegal.

We crave sugar. That should be clue enough. We speak jokingly of being 'sugar junkies' and wanting a 'sugar hit', and jokes are always clues. A substance is addictive when it drives out a natural body function, replacing it with an artificial function on which the body then comes to depend. Smoking, for example, is addictive for two separate reasons. The carbon monoxide in tobacco smoke inhibits the flow of oxygen to the blood, and the nicotine in tobacco inhibits the flow of hormones known as endorphins, the body's natural pain-killers. The craving for cigarettes after giving up smoking is not 'just in the mind'; the body learns to crave carbon monoxide and nicotine.

Likewise, processed sugar overwhelms the body's natural reaction to the sugar within fruit or the starch in vegetables and cereals. Eating processed sugar causes an artificially high blood-sugar level; then, because of the body's defence system, an artificially low blood-sugar level; and so a craving for sugar. As Mr Mars discovered, eating one Mars Bar creates the desire for another Mars Bar.

Table 1. Sugar in Food

It is not easy to avoid eating processed sugar. This table is designed to help you. Foods heavy in processed sugar are included in the first list. The top part, of foods containing more than forty per cent processed sugar, is mostly confectionery; but some sweet breakfast cereals such as Sugar Puffs are not much more than vehicles for sugar. The middle part of the list, of foods containing more than twenty per cent sugar, includes some items tasting fairly savoury or thought of as 'health' foods, such as sweet pickle, rich tea biscuits and packet muesli. The bottom part of the list is a small selection of foods containing more than five per cent sugar. Note the fruit salad: fruits canned in syrup are fifteen to twenty-five per cent processed sugar. Almost all breakfast cereals have added sugar. Soft drinks such as Coca-Cola are basically water, sugar and flavourings. Almost all canned food has added sugar: look at the label.

Sugar supplies nothing but energy. The second list is of foods high in natural sugar, which also contain many nutrients. While honey and dried fruit are both nutritious, it is better to eat them sparingly. Fruit juice has more sugar than the fruit itself, the fibrous content having been removed; prefer the whole fruit.

The body needs sugar for energy, but you do not have to eat food containing sugar. Starch converts to sugar in the body just as readily as dietary sugar. The third list is designed as a means to wean you off processed sugar; it is a selection of dairy products, fruits and vegetables, cereals and other foods containing little or no sugar.

The processed foods always to avoid are sweets and sweet fats, and also processed cereals and vegetables to which sugar, fat or salt has been added. These have little nourishment and often include additives. By contrast the fruit – and some vegetables – that are rich in natural sugars are good for you no matter how much of them you eat. Fruit and vegetables by themselves cannot possibly make you fat; it is only the addition of fat (in the form of cream, perhaps) or of sugar (as in the syrups added to canned fruit) that can be fattening. For most nourishment, fruit and vegetables should be eaten raw.

	per cent		per cent
Sugar (white, brown)	100.0	Muesli (packaged)[1,3]	26.2
Peppermints	100.0	Fruit salad (canned)[3]	25.0
Meringues	95.6	Tomato ketchup[1]	22.9
Boiled sweets	86.9	Ice-cream	22.6
Golden syrup	79.0	Rich tea biscuits	22.3
Drinking chocolate (dry)	73.8	Malt loaf	18.6
Toffees	70.0	Fruit yoghurt[3]	17.9
Jam, marmalade[1]	69.0	Digestive biscuits	16.4
Mars Bar	65.8	All-Bran	15.4
Ribena (undiluted)	60.0	Doughnuts	15.0
Chocolate (plain)	59.5	Jelly (water)	14.2
Chocolate (milk)	56.5	Currant buns	14.0
Sugar Puffs	56.5	Salad cream	13.4
Bounty bar	53.7	Flavoured yoghurt[3]	13.0
Bournvita (dry)	52.0	Coca-Cola	10.5
Horlicks (dry)	49.4	Lucozade	9.0
Fruit cake	46.7	Rice Krispies	9.0
Wafers (filled)	44.7	Canned sweetcorn[3]	8.9
Chocolate biscuits	43.4	Cornflakes	7.4
Ginger nuts	35.8	Crispbread, Energen	7.4
Jam, treacle tart	33.6	Peanut butter[1]	6.7
Branston pickle[1]	32.6	Weetabix	6.1
Sponge cake	30.5	Orangeade (diluted)	5.6
Rusks (for babies)[2]	30.0	Lemonade (diluted)	5.6
Chocolate digestives	28.5	Baked beans (canned)	5.2

[1] Mass manufactured products. Some small firms make them sugar-free. Jams and pickles made without processed sugar need to be kept in a refrigerator once opened.

[2] Sugar-free rusks and other baby foods are now becoming available. Ask for them.

[3] Including small amount of natural sugar content.

	per cent		per cent
Honey[1]	76.0	Plums, damsons	9.6
Sultanas, raisins	64.5	Figs (fresh)	9.5
Dates (dried)	63.9	Orange juice	9.5
Currants	63.1	Sweet potato (boiled)	9.1
Figs (dried)	52.9	Peaches	9.1
Milk (skimmed, dried)[2]	52.8	Oranges[3]	8.5
Apricots (dried)	43.4	Spring onions	8.5
Prunes (dried)	40.3	Damsons (stewed)	8.1
Milk (dried)[2]	39.4	Tangerines	8.0
Prunes (stewed)	20.4	Horseradish (raw)	7.3
Bananas	16.2	Chestnuts	7.0
Lychees (raw)	16.0	Apricots (raw)	6.7
Grapes, white[3]	15.3	Blackcurrants	6.6
Mangoes	15.3	Coconut (dessicated)	6.4
Grapes, black[3]	13.0	Blackberries	6.4
Apple juice	13.0	Strawberries	6.2
Nectarines	12.4	Passion fruit	6.2
Cherries	11.9	Apricots (stewed)	5.6
Apples (raw)[3]	11.8	Raspberries	5.6
Greengages	11.8	Carrots (raw)	5.4
Pineapple[3]	11.6	Grapefruit[3]	5.3
Pomegranates (juice)	11.6	Melons	5.3
Pears[3]	10.6	Onion (raw)	5.2
Onions (fried)	10.1	Chick peas, dahl	5.2
Beetroot (cooked)	9.9	Plums (stewed)	5.2

[1] Honey has nutrients but in a sense is refined (by bees).
[2] Lactose.
[3] Juice from these fruits has 1 to 2 per cent more sugar

	per cent		per cent
Fresh milk[1]	4.7	Cucumbers	1.8
Natural yoghurt[1]	4.6	Corn on the cob	1.7
Leeks (boiled)	4.6	Brussels sprouts	1.6
Almonds	4.3	Puffed wheat	1.5
Carrots (boiled)	4.2	Butter beans	1.5
Coconut	3.7	Runner beans	1.3
Peas (canned)[2]	3.6	Marrow	1.3
Loganberries	3.4	Lettuce	1.2
Crispbread, Ryvita[2]	3.2	Spinach	1.2
Tomato juice	3.2	Celery	1.2
Lemons	3.2	Pastry	1.0
Peanuts	3.1	Cauliflower	0.8
Aubergines	2.9	Lentils	0.8
Gooseberries (stewed)	2.9	Spaghetti, pastas	0.8
Tomatoes	2.8	Potatoes	0.6
Parsnips (boiled)	2.7	Watercress	0.6
Tomato soup[2]	2.6	Shredded wheat	0.4
Vegetable soup[2]	2.5	Olives	Trace
Water biscuits	2.3	Rice	Trace
Instant potato[2]	2.2	Porridge	Trace
White cabbage (boiled)	2.2	Tea	Trace
White bread, rolls[2]	2.0	Artichokes	0
Wholewheat bread	2.0	Mushrooms	0
Peas (fresh)	1.8	Meat, fish	0
Avocado pears	1.8	Marmite	0

[1] Lactose. Yoghurt also has a little galactose.
[2] Processed sugar.

Chief source of information: *McCance and Widdowson's The Composition of Foods* edited by A A Paul and D A T Southgate (HMSO 1978).

CHAPTER FOUR

Swallow It Whole

The word 'health' in English is based on an Anglo-Saxon
word 'hale' meaning 'whole': that is, to be healthy is to be
whole. Likewise, the English 'holy' is based on the same
root as 'whole'. All of this indicates that man has sensed
always that wholeness or integrity is an absolute necessity
to make life worth living.
DAVID BOHM
Wholeness and the Implicate Order

We always had plenty, our children never cried from
hunger, neither were our people in want. The rapids of
Rock River furnished us with an abundance of excellent
fish, and the land being very fertile never failed to produce
good crops of corn, beans, pumpkins, and squashes. If a
prophet had come to our village in those days and told us
that the things were to take place which have since come
to pass, none of our people would have believed him.
BLACK HAWK, CHIEF OF THE SOUK AND FOX
in *Touch the Earth*, by T C McLuhan

More dieting memoirs

In my dieting days, I carried around a leaflet called the
'Unit Eating Guide' whose introduction promised:

An evolutionary approach . . . to the problem of correct
eating. No longer will you be able to say you feel hungry. This
is because a very wide variety of foods can be freely taken at
any time.

Ah! Magic! A diet that didn't involve cutting calories! No
wonder I picked it up. The principle of this system was to

106

concentrate the mind of the dieter on the monster, carbohydrate: 'Keep your carbohydrate consumption down to a low level by taking little of the carbohydrate foods, but as much as you like of the non-carbohydrate foods.'

It was a handy little guide; it listed foods in three groups. Group A was 'eat as much as you like'. It included:

Duck	Cockles	Butter	Cabbage
Black pudding	Cod	Cream cheese	Courgettes
Faggots	Flathead	Processed cheese	Okra
Lard	Jewfish	Cream	Olives
Liver paste	Leather jacket	Margarine	Pumpkin
Suet	Oysters	Cooking oil	Ginger
Tripe	Pollack	Salad oil	Gravy

Group C was printed on red paper. Looking at the leaflet now, I well recall the feelings I had as I peered down the list of the foods which, I was being led to believe, were making me into Michelin Man. 'Danger! Avoid if possible!' was printed on top of this list, rather like the road signs that warn you of falling rocks. The list of baddies included:

Ale	Flour	Macaroni	Spaghetti
All-Bran	Fructose	Oatmeal	Sugar
Bread (brown)	Gin	Plum pudding	Taro
Bread (white)	Grapes	Port	Teff
Cereals	Honey	Potato	Toffees
Bun	Horlicks	Ryvita	Vermicelli
Chocolate	Ice-cream	Sago	Yam

There was a time when I knew these lists more or less off by heart. Their alphabeticisation did hold a certain appeal. Meals of toffees, tonic water, treacle and vermicelli were Out. Menus of garfish, groper, gurnet and haddock were In; as were schnapper, seaslugs, shrimps and skate, or mayonnaise, mustard, pepper and pickles. I wondered, eyeing the oysters in the fishmongers, which fish was the leather jacket. I believed that if, in a cafe, I was told, 'Sorry, love, taro and teff are off,' I was missing nothing that would do me any good.

'One thing you will notice from the examples we have

given, the foods you can eat are quite straightforward ordinary foods, and you can eat them whenever you like,' said the guide. The main warning in the introduction was against the red foods in group C. These were, it said, 'foods that are rich in carbohydrate, and don't contain much in the way of nutrients'. The guide was put out in 1972.

The confusion of starch with sugar

Dr Irwin Stillman's *Doctor's Quick Weight Loss Diet* was popular at about the same time. One of the diets he recommends is the 'HF-HP' diet. 'The usual basic restriction at its strongest may be summed up in one sentence: don't touch carbohydrates, sugar, salt, fruits, cereals, bread, rice, potatoes, alcohol.'

Not only don't eat or drink – don't touch. The inference was not only that carbohydrates made you fat but that they could give you typhoid. Richard Mackarness, a psychiatrist, wrote *Eat Fat and Grow Slim* which, its publishers claim, has sold over a million copies. While warning against sugar and refined foods, Mackarness says:

> Try to develop a carbohydrate alarm system, so that whenever you are confronted with a food which does or even *might* contain carbohydrate, a little bell goes off in your head and you avoid the temptation to eat it.

Unclean! Unclean! 'The first thing to realise', writes Dr Mackarness 'is that it is carbohydrate (starch and sugar) and carbohydrate only, which fattens fat people.'

The Consumers' Association is also enthusiastic about low-carbohydrate diets, as an alternative to diets that cut calories. In *Which? Way to Slim*, published in 1978, the authors say:

> The foods which are richest in carbohydrate are, on the whole, the ones which are poorest in proteins, vitamins and minerals ... The low carbohydrate diet is therefore particularly suitable for growing children.

108

Much like my 'Unit Eating Guide' and Dr Mackarness, *Which?* says of carbohydrate-rich food: 'Think of it as a traffic light. The red light means STOP for the things to avoid . . .' And the list includes bread, breakfast cereals, biscuits, flour, honey, nuts, potatoes, spaghetti, sugar and sweets. In the section on staying slim after following the low-carbohydrate method, *Which?* lets the slimmer-pilgrim know that she is on a long, stony road. A cartoon shows a housewife polishing a sideboard, eyeing a plate of biscuits with a red 'X' through them. The text says:

> By following the low-carbohydrate method, you had to cut right down on sweet and starchy foods. If you have managed to do this successfully while you were losing weight, you may well be happy never to see a chocolate or potato again. Your only danger then would be eating too much protein and fat which would supply too many calories.

The basic message, though, is that the baddies are sugar and starch, bracketed together as carbohydrates.

Vogue magazine has followed the same line for many years. In the 1960s it said: 'The simplest do-it-yourself answer is – we're sorry to say – some kind of crash diet. It's human nature to want quick results so, for quick returns, cut out starch and sugar.'

In 1966 *Vogue* produced a Peanut Diet, 'devised by one of Britain's leading nutrition consultants'. 'Forbidden foods include everything made with flour or cornflour, root vegetables, peas, beans, cereals, pastas, all sugar, sweets, sweetened drinks.' The dieter is told to replace one of the main meals of the day with 2 oz of peanuts (with salt) and also an orange.

The *Vogue Book of Diets and Exercise,* published in 1980, lists various low-carbohydrate diets, including one recommended by Edgar S Gordon, Professor of Medicine at the University of Wisconsin; one created for the late Aga Khan (a man not noted for a slim figure); and one by Robert Atkins, of *Dr Atkins' Diet Revolution* and *Dr Atkins' Nutrition Breakthrough*. No peanuts, says Dr Atkins. And, in the Jove-like style he shares with Dr Stillman, Dr Tarnower and all the most effective snake-oil salesmen, prophetic, fatherly, threatening, he says:

Super Don'ts. Put these out of your life (and your recipes). Bread, cereal, corn, ice-cream, ketchup, macaroni, milk, potatoes, pulse vegetables, rice, spaghetti, sugar, sweets/chewing gum, water biscuits. Note: one piece of chewing gum can spoil the whole chemical balance.

Until Audrey Eyton's *F-Plan Diet*, the best-selling diet book in Great Britain was Professor John Yudkin's *This Slimming Business*, first published in 1958. Yudkin is best known professionally for his hostility to processed sugar. But in his writings for the general public, dieters in particular, this hostility has been extended to all carbohydrates. He is an author and writer of numerous articles (sometimes under a *nom de plume*) for periodicals, and a nutrition consultant; and he has probably done more than any other nutritionist to have us believe that carbohydrates are, for the slimmer, the villain.

Yudkin's theory of nutrition is that the food eaten by our hunter-gatherer ancestors was meat, fish, roots, berries, fruit, leaves, rich in protein and also fat, but including little carbohydrate. On this theory, he gives us a model to follow, a 'Stone Age Diet': 'The nearer we get to man's hunting and food gathering diet, the more likely we are to be well-nourished, and the more we can depend on our instinctive choice.' Yudkin sees agriculture as a snare. The discovery of cereals encouraged settlement and the beginning of civilisation. The agriculturist's food is chiefly composed of carbohydrate and contains less protein and fat than that of the hunter-gatherer. And, Yudkin concludes, in a passage which in effect provides the intellectual underpinning for all low-carbohydrate diets: 'My theory is that this is the fundamental fault with the diets of civilisation.' He then goes on to set out his system of 'carbohydrate units', explaining that all the dieter need do is memorise a long list of carbohydrate-rich foods and, on the whole, avoid them.

My 'Unit Eating Guide' also used the carbohydrate unit system. I got it from a doctor who prescribed the slimming drug 'Ponderax' (fenfluramine) for me. The Guide is given out, free, to doctors, world-wide, by Servier Laboratories, manufacturers of Ponderax, claimed to be a slimming drug that is not addictive. Servier estimate that they have produced 250,000 copies of the Guide, which is now in wall-chart form. Servier's nutritional consultant is Professor John Yudkin.

Not so much is heard nowadays of low-carbohydrate diets. One reason is that late in his career Yudkin changed his view, and came to acknowledge that starch should not be confused with sugar, as he and two or three generations of Western nutritionists had done. But this confusion suits a powerful section of industry. The Health Education Council commissioned Aubrey Sheiham, an authority on dental disease, to write a report on the information the British public receives about sugar. This report, after completion, was semi-suppressed after pressure was applied by representatives of the sugar industry. The report, *Sweet Nothings* (co-written by Helena Sheiham and Alison Quick) shows that the British public is still being confused about starch and sugar. For example, the British Medical Association's *You and Your Baby*, produced for mothers in 1977, says 'Do eat sensibly. It means eating little carbohydrate.' Boots produced a leaflet for expectant mothers in 1975. It says: 'Potatoes, bread, sugar, cakes and biscuits are carbohydrates. They provide energy and warmth, but should only be taken sparingly.'

Professor Yudkin is also consultant to the National Dairy Council, whose *Keeping Fit in Retirement* says: 'If you want to lose some weight, cut out or reduce some of the "starchy" foods you eat. These are bread, cakes, pastry, sugar, jam, rice, biscuits, cereals and potatoes.'

Ironically, given Yudkin's hostility to processed sugar, his old argument that starch and sugar are equally objectionable is turned on its head by the sugar manufacturers, who argue that sugar and starch are equally desirable. The British Sugar Bureau, the publicity organisation for Tate and Lyle and British Sugar, published *Questions and Answers on Sugar* in 1977, circulating it free to NHS and private doctors, to doctors and surgeons in hospitals, to health education officers, 1224 registered dieticians and 600 medical correspondents of the national press and women's magazines. I first came across it on the shelves of the Health Education Council's library. *Questions and Answers* says that processed sugar is a carbohydrate which is easily absorbed and enables the body to replace lost energy quickly. This property is appreciated by athletes, sportsmen, busy mothers and active growing children . . . Our calorie needs are provided by balanced meals containing protein, carbohydrates, including starches and sugars, and fats. When weight reduction is indicated most dieticians support an overall reduction in food intake.

Everybody who has been on a low-carbohydrate diet will recognise the language used to make the dieter conform. 'Danger!' 'Try to develop a carbohydrate alarm system.' 'Think of it as a traffic light.' '. . . the whole chemical balance'. 'Should be taken only sparingly.' The metaphors and images buzz around the brain of the bemused dieter, who is invited to think of carbohydrates as an abyss, a burglar, oncoming traffic, a toxin, or a medicine. Always, though, the dieter is told to distrust his or her own body; and women are especially susceptible to this message.

British housewives were asked in a survey to name the foods that should be avoided when slimming. The eight foods most often named were:

Potatoes	62%	Starches	22%
Bread	55%	Sweets	16%
Sugar	31%	Fat	10%
Cakes	25%	Carbohydrate	7%

Biscuits, pastry, fried food and butter came further down the list. In the minds of slimmers and would-be slimmers sugars and starches are mingled together. For the last twenty years and more, British mothers, children, dieters, pensioners, doctors, dieticians, nutritionists, health educators, nurses, journalists, and readers of newspapers, magazines and books have been taught, systematically, to think of carbohydrates as bad food and to think of sugars and starches therefore as equally bad. In its publicity the sugar industry reinforces this message, proposing that sugars and starches are equally good.

The medical revolution for the 1980s

All this is changing now, and the change is radical. In

February 1977 a committee of the United States Senate, chaired by Senator George McGovern, published a report, *Dietary Goals For The United States*. Senator McGovern's preliminary statement sets the tone of a report which, more than any other single influence, is changing the food habits of Americans:

> The simple fact is that our diets have changed radically within the last fifty years, with great and often very harmful effects on our health . . . Too much fat, too much sugar or salt, can be and are linked directly to heart disease, cancer, obesity and stroke, among other killer diseases. In all, six of the ten leading causes of death in the United States have been linked to our diet. Those of us within Government have an obligation to acknowledge this.

The report begins by making the sharpest possible distinction between starch and sugar. It points out that processed foods saturated with sugar, fat and salt are massively advertised, whereas foods rich in starch – whole grains and vegetables – are rarely advertised. In less than thirty years, the consumption of grain, vegetables and fruits has dropped dramatically.

The report makes a sharp distinction between starch and sugar, on health grounds. It points out that starchy foods like cereals and vegetables are rich in vitamins and minerals (micronutrients), as is fruit:

> Increased consumption of fruit, vegetables and whole grains is also important with respect to supplying adequate amounts of micronutrients, vitamins and minerals. This is particularly important for those who are limiting their food intake to control weight or save money. For many people consumption may be reaching a critical level below which it may be difficult to obtain adequate levels of micronutrients.

The report also shows that consumption of whole foods, starchy foods in particular, has dropped dramatically since the last World War, and that sugar, together with fat, is a poor source of nourishment. Suddenly, in America, the doctors and scientists who knew the vital importance of whole food, and knew what was wrong with sugar, together with fat and salt, were no longer lonely voices:

113

they had the American government behind them. The US Dietary Goals proposed that consumption of starchy foods be doubled (from a figure of twenty-two per cent of total energy intake, to forty to forty-five per cent) and that the consumption of sugar be sharply cut (from twenty-four per cent of energy intake, to fifteen per cent):

	Total energy intake %	
	US 1977	McGovern Goal
Protein	12	12
Fat	42	30
Starch	22	40 – 45
Sugar	24	15
Total	100	100

The report also emphasises that, completely contrary to what has been stated in so many dieting books, starchy foods are not fattening. Earlier in this book the twenty-three young men of Galway who lost weight on Dr Denis Burkitt's potato diet were mentioned. The McGovern report points out that bread, too, is not fattening. Quite the reverse:

> Contrary to what most people think, bread in large amounts is an ideal food in a weight reducing programme . . . Slightly overweight young men lost weight in a painless and practically effortless manner when they included twelve slices of bread a day in their programme. The bread was eaten with their meals. As a result, they became satiated before they consumed their usual quota of calories.

The young men were asked to go easy on sugar and fats; otherwise, they could eat what they liked – provided that they ate the bread. In eight weeks they lost an average of over twelve pounds.

In 1983 the Royal College of Physicians of London, in their report on obesity, likewise made a clear distinction between starch and sugar, and, again, emphasised that starchy foods are not fattening:

> The public and many in the medical profession have come to consider dietary carbohydrates as being particularly

114

> conducive to weight gain and the development of obesity, no distinction being made between sucrose (sugar) and starch as sources of dietary carbohydrate

and, referring to starches, the report went on to say that 'low carbohydrate diets are inappropriate on general nutritional grounds.'

The Royal College agree with the McGovern committee that fat intake should be reduced to thirty per cent of total calories. With processed sugar they go a little further, recommending that we should eat half the amount we now eat.

In the last decade or so, countries all over the developed world have been issuing recommendations along the same lines. The story behind this radical new view of the relationship between the food we eat, and obesity, health and disease, is the story of a group of British doctors who are having the impact on medicine that Darwin had on science and Keynes had on economics.

Whole food: the founding doctors

These doctors, with their followers, have demonstrated beyond all reasonable doubt that the diseases that most of us suffer and die from in the West (and which are – often ineffectively – treated by the medicine of drugs and surgery) are caused, above all other causes, by what we eat and what we do not eat. These non-infectious, Western diseases can, therefore, be prevented.

Between now and the end of the century, Western medicine will experience the biggest change ever in its history: towards prevention. This movement will be encouraged by citizens who are appalled by the effects of drugs and who, by taking responsibility for themselves, will encourage doctors to practise the medicine of health rather than illness. It will require massive re-allocations of money; it is estimated that only one per cent of total health expenditure in Britain is devoted to the prevention of disease. And above all, it will require government and industry to work together with a will. Senator Charles Percy of the McGovern committee, had this to say:

Without government and industry commitment to good nutrition, the American people will continue to eat themselves to bad health . . . Our national health depends on how well and how quickly government and industry respond.

The same is true in Britain.

The value of whole food

So far the thesis of this book could be said to amount to two 'don'ts'. If you want to lose fat, and if you want to gain health, do not go on a diet, and do not eat processed food, especially sugar. The rest of this chapter is concerned with good food – with the unprocessed, starchy foods so long wrongly blamed as a cause of fatness, so long condemned as having little nourishment; now rightly championed as the staff of life.

T L Cleave's reputation now, is above all that of the doctor who has exposed the role of processed sugar in obesity and disease. But Cleave always, at the same time, advocated whole, starchy foods. He is opposed to the spoonful of sugar; he is in favour of the apple:

> It is perfectly true that the calories in, for example an apple, are much the same as those in a teaspoonful of sugar, and therefore at first sight the danger in cases of obesity would appear to be the same in each. But there is an enormous difference between the two in one vital respect – the amount a person needs to consume of each before the appetite is appeased. A person may over-consume sugar very easily – but not apples.

For Cleave the difference between eating processed sugar and eating apples (including natural sugar) is the one between craving and satisfaction, between obesity and no obesity.

Since Cleave began his pioneering work, other British doctors, with him, emphasised not only the dangers of processed sugar but also – and to a considerable extent this is the other side of the same coin – the benefits of dietary fibre. Fibre is that part of food derived from the cellular walls of plants such as sugar cane. In effect it is the skeleton of the plant. It is of course discarded in the refining process. Humans digest little of it, and until recently therefore nutritionists and doctors assumed that fibre had no value as food.

The identification of the value of dietary fibre has been principally a British achievement, a result, as Dr Hugh Trowell has explained to me, of the British 'having colonies where doctors could study the changing incidence of disease in time and in place and in various groups over a period of several years. History and geography favoured us.'

Sir Robert McCarrison was Director of Research on Nutrition in India, then part of the British Empire, in the 1920s. He was impressed by the superb health and physique of people of the state of Hunza in northernmost India, 'whose sole food to this day consists of grains, vegetables, and fruits, with a certain amount of milk and butter, and meat only on feast days'. Although they dwelt in primitive and harsh conditions, the Hunza in McCarrison's day were long-lived, and their illnesses were wholly unconnected with food. By contrast, McCarrison deplored the state of health of European people, fed on processed food. 'Green vegetables are scanty, and such as there are, are often cooked to the point of almost complete extraction of their vitamin content and salts. White bread has largely replaced wholewheat bread.' And he noted that a drop in infant and adult mortality accompanied the national canteens established in Belgium during the First World War, and the consumption of large quantities of whole cereals and potatoes in Denmark during the same war. Ironically, shortages forced the Danes to eat this healthy food; in peacetime cattle and swine ate the cereals and potatoes.

In his book *Nutrition and Health*, McCarrison also quoted studies by Dr G E Friend, of special interest to me because Friend was the doctor – before my time – at my own school, Christ's Hospital. I well remember, in the 1950s, eating Prewett's wholewheat and 'squashed fly' biscuits (the latter named after the dried fruit they contained), the remnants of the doctor's campaign against refined food. Alas, the boys of my generation tended to flick Mr Prewett's good food at each other, like miniature frisbees. They were effective missiles. We preferred to eat sugary biscuits from our tuck lockers, having no idea of Dr Friend's principles: 'The deficiency of white bread in Vitamin B_1 is one of the most serious dietary deficiencies to which our populations are being subjected.'

Health in black Africa and during wars

Dr Alec Walker, who left Great Britain for South Africa in 1938, has extended McCarrison's work. Dr Walker has studied the changes in eating habits and disease patterns in black Africans who have moved from rural to urban areas and in Indians moving from rural India to urban South Africa. He has found that the move into urban areas reduces the life expectancy of middle-aged Africans and Indians. In 1974 he reported that the expectation of life of South African blacks aged fifty exceeded that of whites of the same age. In rural India people of fifty usually died of infectious diseases and had over fourteen per cent chance of reaching the age of seventy; in South Africa they usually died of coronary heart disease, strokes, cancer or diabetes and had only a nine per cent chance of reaching seventy. At an older age the differences are even more remarkable: 'allowing for differences in population numbers, there are at least twenty times more Bantu over 100 years old than whites.'

Dr Denis Burkitt, who worked for thirty years as a surgeon in East Africa, also observed that Africans living in rural areas did not get fat:

> In the 1920s doctors in East Africa reported that almost every African was slim. Even the soldiers who were liberally fed with traditional African food rarely appeared obese. In contrast urban Africans are commonly obese today and some of the overweight rulers are familiar figures on news media.

Like Dr Burkitt, Dr Walker became convinced that rural Africans and Indians who moved to urban areas began to suffer from obesity, and die from Western diseases, because their eating habits changed. Their traditional food, like the traditional food of virtually everybody

118

in the world before the spread of industrialisation in the West, was mainly composed of whole grain, rich in starch, protein fibre and other nutrients, lightly processed and lightly – if at all – cooked, together with vegetables and fruit. But in the urban areas they ate sugar and fat instead of cereal, and fewer vegetables. The dramatic difference was the virtual elimination of fibre.

Dr Hugh Trowell was the first person to identify 'Western diseases' as such. He worked in the same large teaching hospital in Uganda as Dr Burkitt. His book *Non-infectious Diseases in Africa*, proposing that fibre gives protection against various diseases of the lower gut and bowel, was published in 1960; and sold twenty-seven copies in its first year. Undaunted, Trowell, with Burkitt, later identified seventeen diseases of previously uncertain origin that are common in the West and sent the list to thirty-four doctors working in teaching hospitals all over the world. Their response confirmed that these diseases were rare among hunter-gatherers, uncommon among peasants, but common among people with Western food habits.

Dr Cleave was independently accumulating his own evidence against processed sugar and in favour of unprocessed cereal. In the Second World War, enemy attacks on Allied convoys reduced supplies of wheat to Great Britain from the USA. The government therefore stipulated that bread should contain much more of the whole wheat. The 'National Loaf' was the staple food from 1941 to 1954, when restrictions were lifted and the white loaf most people eat today was introduced. Cleave points out that between 1941 and 1954 mortality from diabetes fell by fifty-four per cent, a finding similar to Sir Robert McCarrison's in the previous war.

The people of Singapore, faced with acute food shortages before the island fell to the Japanese in 1942, were compelled by the British authorities to eat whole, brown rice, simply because the processing and polishing of rice resulted in thirty out of every 100 tons of whole grain being discarded. After one year of this regime infant mortality fell by half.

Cleave made two more remarkable discoveries in the

119

Second World War. His brother, Surgeon-Captain Hugh Cleave, was a prisoner of war of the Japanese and the surgeon in charge of British prisoners in Hong Kong and later in Tokyo. British prisoners who worked on the Burma railway were fed whole, brown rice and bran normally fed to swine. They did not suffer from ulcers of the stomach and gut. In Hong Kong, prisoners were fed processed white rice; ulcers were common. The same prisoners were then transferred to Tokyo and fed brown rice; the ulcers vanished. Ulcers are often blamed on stress. But the ulcer-free prisoners in Tokyo were being held in a city that was largely destroyed by American bombing.

Cleave himself corresponded extensively with Germans who served and were made prisoner on the Russian Front. To the astonishment of German doctors in the front line, the closer their soldiers came to the Russians in the Stalingrad campaign, and the more anxiety, cold and fatigue they suffered, the fewer ulcers they had. The reason, Cleave came to realise, was that over-extended supply lines forced the soldiers to forage for food. They ate frozen raw vegetables, turnips in particular, and sour wholemeal bread. One ex-prisoner wrote to Cleave:

> Our bread in the Russian camps did not consist of refined flour, but of unrefined wheat, rye, barley or maize, with frequently up to twenty per cent of peas, beans or soya bean. We were fed the Russian way. Cabbage soup played a dominant part.

While in captivity the Germans ate little animal protein, animal fat or processed sugar. They had no ulcers. After repatriation to Germany, many of those who had ulcers before the Russian campaign suffered relapses.

More recently, in a study of 337 middle-aged men in London, Professor J N (Jerry) Morris of the London School of Hygiene and Tropical Medicine found that men least subject to certain types of heart disease were those who ate most wholewheat bread and breakfast cereal, most vegetable (as opposed to animal) fat, and whose energy intake from food was highest. The men most liable to heart attacks ate the least amount of starchy food.

120

During the 1970s, leading doctors established that whole starchy food, with its fibre, is a protection against those diseases that are caused by eating processed sugary food. For many years diabetics, rather like dieters, were told to avoid all carbohydrates. Now diabetics are told to avoid only sugars, and to eat large quantities of whole starchy food. Likewise, whole foods are a valuable means to improve the quality of the blood and so reduce the risk of heart attacks; and they also prevent gallstones. Again, the bulk of whole foods is more satisfying than concentrated processed foods, and so whole foods protect against obesity. Whether you are healthy, fit, fat, suffering from various Western diseases or at risk from them, or just want to gain a sense of well-being, the story is the same: eat whole food.

The value of fibre

Dietary fibre is that part of plants which is not digested by the small intestine. Fibre itself is essentially not a nutrient, but a package within which nutrients are contained. Foods that have fibre processed out of them, lose nourishment with the fibre. This is why whole foods including fibre are good for us, and processed foods, especially sugar, without fibre and with little or no nourishment, are bad for us.

Whole foods travel through the upper alimentary tract at a natural speed – relatively slowly. The fibre that binds the food allows its nutrients to be released into the bloodstream gradually, not in a rush. This is why starch (in the form of wholewheat bread, say) raises the blood-sugar level, but at a natural speed; whereas sugar (in the form of candy or a soft drink, say) is liable to provoke an insulin response, with the eventual consequence of obesity, diabetes or heart disease. Likewise, the natural sugars in fruit are released slowly into the blood stream. (Dr Kenneth Heaton has established that fruit juices, and even purees, can provoke an insulin response; the whole fruit is to be preferred).

The bulk of whole food gives the muscles of the

121

intestines the work they are designed to do. The passage of fibre-rich food through the lower alimentary tract is comparatively faster. The fibre absorbs acids in the large bowel which, without the presence of fibre, become toxic, cause irritation, and eventually the risk of cancer. With fibre, stools are soft, large, and easily evacuated. People who eat plenty of whole starchy food do not get constipated; and fibre-rich food protects against piles, irritable bowels, and more serious conditions such as varicose veins, hernias, diverticular disease (rupture of the lower gut) and cancer of the large bowel, all caused by pressure, irritation or poisoning in the lower gut.

The culmination of the work of Cleave, Trowell, Burkitt and their colleagues and followers was the publication, in 1980, of the Royal College of Physicians' report *Medical Aspects of Dietary Fibre* which, with some qualifications, supported their views. Nutrition is once again becoming central to medicine, as it was since the foundation of medicine until its recent domination by machines, money and drugs.

Britain: the backward nation

As I proceeded with the research for the first edition of this book, and its thesis developed, the same question kept on nagging at me. Given that all this is true, why hadn't I heard it already? When I read the McGovern report, and the Royal College of Physicians' reports on dietary fibre and then on obesity – the second of which was published as I was writing the book – I realised that the crucial importance of whole food to health, and the causal relationship between processed food and disease, including overweight and obesity, were not ideas confined to 'health food' enthusiasts. Only when I had done a lot of research for the book, did I have a clear idea of the relationship between food and health. I had been in the dark. It was only after the first edition of the book was published that I discovered, in the course of my work for *The Sunday Times*, that I, in common with every other British citizen, had been kept in the dark.

For the answer to the question 'if all this is true, why

haven't I heard it already?' is 'in whose interests is it to tell you the truth?' This is not how a democracy is supposed to work but, certainly as far as food and health is concerned, it is how things are in Britain. For the story that unfolded in *The Sunday Times* was described by one doctor as the biggest scandal in British public health since the days, 140 years ago, when public officials and private companies combined to conceal the evidence that cholera is a water-borne disease.

In 1979 the relevant government department, of health (the DHSS) set up a National Advisory Committee on Nutrition Education (which became known as NACNE). Partners in NACNE were the DHSS-funded Health Education Council, and the food industry-funded British Nutrition Foundation. One of the motives behind the setting up of NACNE was a statement made by Sir Keith Joseph, then the politician responsible for the DHSS, in 1973, to the effect that the British public was muddled about what is good food and what is bad food, and should be guided. Chairman of NACNE was Professor J N Morris. In 1980 Professor Morris asked a leading nutritionist who is also a doctor of medicine, Professor Philip James, to prepare a report specifically on what guidelines the British public should follow in choosing what food to eat.

Professor James was asked to gather together a group of doctors, scientists and nutritionists to help him prepare the report; which he did. In 1981 he produced a report whose conclusions were broadly speaking those of the McGovern report, and for the same reasons. The James report stated that the food we now eat in Britain is the main single cause of the diseases that most of us suffer and die from, and that we should, to ensure health, cut down the amount of fat, salt – and sugar – that we eat. And, like the McGovern report, the James report specified how much less of each we should eat.

One of the members of the NACNE main committee, to whom Professor James reported, was a member of the staff of the Food and Drinks Industries Council, the lobby organisation for the British food and drinks industry. He objected to the James report. So did the representatives of the British Nutrition Foundation. And so did the Department of Health, which effectively controlled the

NACNE committee, and which in turn is influenced by the Ministry of Agriculture, Fisheries and Food, which protects the British farmers and food industry.

On three occasions Professor James revised his report, between 1980 and April 1983. It was rejected again and again. The outrage that the behaviour of the public officials and private companies represented on NACNE had meanwhile caused among doctors, scientists and nutritionists in the know, was so intense that I was told the full story, which I started to publish in *The Sunday Times* in July 1983. Subsequently, under pressure from the doctor's journal *The Lancet*, and from the great majority of members of the NACNE committee that agreed with Professor James, it was agreed that the Health Education Council should issue the James report, as a 'discussion document'. What this means, is that the report could no longer be kept secret. But the Department of Health disowned it; so there is no pressure on the British farmers and food industry to move towards the production and distribution of healthy food.

Meanwhile, the rate of heart attacks has decreased in the United States by over twenty-five per cent in the last fifteen years; whereas the rate of heart attacks in Britain has not significantly decreased: and Scotland and Northern Ireland now have the highest rate of heart attacks in the world, with England and Wales not far behind. In America, people have been changing their food habits; all the more so, as a result of the publication of the McGovern report. In Britain nothing has happened.

Farmers, food manufacturers and retailers, have a responsibility to make and to sell us good food, whether or not they are encouraged to do so by government. Fortunately, Britain has a special tradition, in that food businessmen of the most remarkable skill, like the Cadburys, the Rowntrees, the Marks (of Marks and Spencer) and the Sainsburys, have combined ability to make money, with a commitment to the health and welfare of their fellow citizens. The movement towards good health by means of good food, in Britain, is not likely to be initiated by government. Enlightened businessmen could take the lead. It would be pleasant if this began during the lifetimes of some of those British doctors who realised the cause of Western diseases.

Fibre: healthy, or a slimming aid?

Audrey Eyton's *F-Plan Diet* has publicised fibre as a slimming aid. It is true that fibre-rich food is liable to be more satisfying than processed food. One study has shown that wholewheat bread is more satisfying than white bread, for example. Given the choice and asked to eat until they felt full, ten out of twelve people ate more white bread than wholewheat bread. Including the energy value of the butter spread on the bread, those who ate the wholewheat bread were satisfied with 665 calories on average; those who ate the white bread – with less fibre and a lot less nourishment in it – went on to eat 825 calories.

So there is something in what Mrs Eyton says. The food she recommends in the *F-Plan Diet* is, together with that stipulated by American nutritionist Nathan Pritikin as part of his diet and exercise programmes, more healthy than that of other popular diet regimes.

There is a danger, though, that dietary fibre will gain the status of a sort of medicine. As an example, in response to a feature I wrote for *The Sunday Times* in July 1983 pointing out the value of fibre in whole food, 'Vita-Fibre', a manufacturer of pills said to be fibrous, purchased a £9000 advertisement. (I never learned how a pill can be fibrous: perhaps Vita-Fibre unfolds in the gut, like those little Japanese novelty items that swell into dragons, placed in water). As with vitamins and minerals, fibre is a natural part of whole food. It would be a disaster if it became perceived as a supplement, to be sprinkled on top of processed food from which fibre – together with vitamins and minerals, and other nourishment – has been removed. Dr Denis Burkitt has put the point in a letter to me. 'The right approach is a healthy diet, not a poor diet plus pills.'

Another reason to stay away from fibre supplements, and to prefer whole food, is that dietary fibre is not one simple substance. Rather like the B complex of vitamins, dietary fibre is a whole series of substances, part of

125

different types of whole food, with different functions in the body. The pentoses, for example, are one part of fibre, notably found in cereals, that increase the bulk of stools. People who eat bran or feed it to horses are aware of the effect of pentoses. Other components of fibre are lignin, pectin and gum. They have different properties. Pectin, for example, present in apples, is good for the blood. The best policy is to eat a wide range of fresh, whole cereals, vegetables, and also fruit.

Unfortunately, Audrey Eyton also recommends processed foods. Heinz baked beans, for example, are high in fibre but also contain over five per cent processed sugar. Prefer beans baked at home. Again, Kelloggs All-Bran contains well over fifteen per cent processed sugar. For breakfast cereals, prefer shredded wheat, or sugar-free muesli, eaten with plain yoghurt and fruit.

It is a pity that Mrs Eyton's recipes do not avoid processed food. Above all, the fault of the *F-Plan* is that her regimes, of 1000 – 1500 calories, cannot contain enough nourishment. But anyone who eats whole food versions of *F-Plan* recipes, eats around twice as much the amounts of food stipulated, and at the same time takes plenty of the type of exercise recommended in the next chapter ('More Air! More Air!') will gradually and reliably lose fat and gain health.

The value of cereals

The best food on earth is eaten by people who grow and eat their own food: peasants. In 1973 the Food and Agriculture Organisation (FAO) and the World Health Organisation (WHO) jointly published the results of a massive survey by Dr J Périssé, an FAO expert, into eating habits in eighty-five countries. In the light of the discoveries by Cleave, Burkitt, Trowell and the other doctors, the results of the FAO survey have become a key to our new understanding of what is healthy food.

The survey divided the eighty-five countries into four groups. The countries with least money, with 760 million inhabitants, had an average income per head per year of less than $100. The countries with most money, including the Western nations, had an income of $600 – $2600 per head per year. The two intermediate groups of countries, with 605 million inhabitants between them, had an average income of $100 – $600 per head per year.

The eating habits of the countries with least money proved to be profoundly different from those with most money. And the change from a 'poor', or peasant, pattern of eating to a 'rich', or Western, pattern proved to be systematic.

If food is categorised as protein, fat and carbohydrate – the conventional division – then the differences between the poor and the rich countries are remarkable enough. Measured as a percentage of total energy intake, protein consumption in the poor and rich countries was much the same: eleven to twelve per cent. Fat consumption was massively different: twelve per cent in the poor countries rising to over forty per cent in the rich countries (such as Great Britain and the USA). Carbohydrate consumption dropped correspondingly, from about seventy-seven per cent in the poor countries to forty-five per cent in the rich. This was confirmed by the McGovern report on dietary goals for the USA in 1977. (The figures for Britain today are much the same).

But these figures disguise the really massive difference in eating habits. Since the invention of agriculture about 10,000 years ago, cereals, rich in starch and fibre and other nutrients, have been the staple food of mankind. All countries developed a staple grain with which to make bread or an equivalent food: wheat in Europe and North America, corn in South America; rice in the East; and millet, rye, barley and oats elsewhere. Contrary to Professor Yudkin's thesis, it is evident from examination of fossil human teeth that pre-agricultural man was principally not a meat-eater, but a fruit- and plant-eater.

The cultivation of wheat from a hybrid of wild wheat and goat grass encouraged human settlement and, with it, the cultivation of other starchy foods: the pea and bean family (also known as pulses and legumes) and root vegetables (including tubers; notably, in recent times, the potato).

Naturally enough, therefore, the FAO survey showed that the poor nations consume about seventy per cent of their energy from whole carbohydrate foods: cereals and also pulses, legumes and root vegetables. These they eat lightly cooked or uncooked. And almost all the protein and fat eaten comes from these foods, as vegetable protein and vegetable fat. Only a tiny percentage of energy comes from animal protein and fat – about seven per cent in the poorest countries. The percentage of vegetable protein and fat amounts to about sixteen per cent. The remaining seven per cent is processed carbohydrate – mostly sugar, introduced recently. The main difference between these figures, researched in the early 1970s, and now is that consumption of sugar, which is distributed and sold cheaply all over the world nowadays, is steadily rising.

In many countries most people do not get enough to eat. Very many people in the poorest countries are starving, and suffering and dying from deficiency diseases, and from infectious diseases liable to be deadly if the victim is malnourished. And in other countries the land may be bad, the farming policies foolish or, as in any feudal society, the peasants be subject to greedy rulers.

That said, a peasant in a settled society, whose wealth is his land and his produce, may neither need nor use much money, especially in a peasant society whose economy is largely one of barter. A peasant is liable to be classified as 'poor' simply because of using little money; but can in truth be well off. In good times and on good land, a peasant can enjoy plentiful, fresh whole cereals, vegetables and fruit, with meat and fish as occasional treats or in effect as a sauce, and, in the matter of health rather than wealth, be rich.

The life expectancy of Greeks, at the age of forty, is notably higher than that of the British. On holiday in the Greek islands it is easy to know why. One day in 1983, for example, I visited Ioannis, who owns a farm in the mountains of Paros. He walks much of the day. He offers visitors a selection of what he grows: grapes, apples, cherries, walnuts, marrows, peppers, aubergines. He shares his produce with the villagers a couple of miles below; he eats bread ground by the mill overlooking Naxos; drinks wine, eau de vie and cherry brandy made from his own fruit; and may buy meat, fish and cheese. To a Western European it may not be an exciting life; but it's a healthy life.

Western countries have moved from a peasant economy to one dependent on industrialisation, among the consequences of which is processed food. Food is processed not for reasons of health, but for reasons of trade. The food that makes money for industry is food that keeps and travels well; and of all such foods sugar is the chief. Having no life, processed sugar does not rot.

At the same time, the rich countries have the money to grow prodigious quantities of grain. Michel Cépède, a French professor who works for the FAO, has calculated that whereas an inhabitant of the Third World eats somewhat over 400 pounds of cereal a year, British and North American people consume five times as much – nearly a ton of cereal a year – almost all of which is fed to animals raised for food. The amount of cereal actually eaten in Great Britain, North America and other Western countries is not much more than one-third of the amount in the Third World. Only rich countries can afford to breed animals for meat.

Industrialisation brings with it reliance on processed food. In the nineteenth century the people who suffered most from processed food were the working classes in Western cities. Later, malnutrition from processed food spread to other parts of the world, for example to Asians who contracted beri-beri from eating processed, white rice while having no money with which to buy other nutritious food. The least fortunate people in Third World countries are now being converted from peasant economies by the spread of industrialisation; they can only afford processed food. Economic colonialism is sometimes grimly termed 'Coca-colonisation'.

Industrialised people eat sugar and fat

Western nations eat meat and animal products, which they can afford. The FAO figures show just how dramatically different Western food is from that of peasant countries. In the richest countries energy taken from animal protein is about eight per cent of the whole; from animal fat (including dairy produce) about thirty per cent. The total of vegetable protein and fat consumed in the West is about fourteen per cent. The colossal difference between the poor and the rich countries is in carbohydrates: the West eats less than one-third the amount of whole carbohydrate eaten in peasant countries, and this tends to be in the form of vegetables rather than cereals. As a result, the volume of cereal fibre (which provides greater protection against diseases of the gut) eaten in Western countries may be only one-fifth that eaten in peasant countries.

In the rich countries, industrialisation has replaced cereals as a staple food with processed foods, and with meat and dairy produce. Peasant countries affected by industrialisation get the processed food without the meat and dairy produce. Ironically it is the peasant countries with the lowest income per head, where very little processed food is eaten, that give us some guide to the food we need to keep and gain our health. This table shows the contrast between the types of food eaten in peasant and in Western countries:

	Energy consumed (%)	
	Peasant	Western
Vegetable protein	7	4
Animal protein	4	8
Total	11	12
Vegetable fat	9	10
Animal fat	3	30
Total	12	40
Whole carbohydrate	70	22
Processed carbohydrate	7	26
Total	77	48
Total vegetable foods	93	62
Total animal foods	7	38

The conventional division of food is between protein, fat and carbohydrate, with energy value included. This is because these were the first divisions made by food chemists. Later, during this century, vitamins were identified and the value of vitamins and minerals established. So we are taught to think of foods as divided somewhat like a book, into a first part (energy – calories), a second part with three sections (protein, fat and carbohydrate) and then a lot of appendices with odd titles that tend to be skipped (vitamins, minerals). Unless we make a conscious decision not to do so, we are bound to think of food in this way simply because this is how books on nutrition are arranged.

130

Nutritionists and diet doctors, and their readers, are now accustomed to a dialogue (a monologue in the case of dieters, who are expected to keep quiet and obey) in which calories are regarded with suspicion; protein is praised; carbohydrates are condemned (usually); fat is condemned (almost always); vitamins are praised and touted (as a form of medicine); and, now, fibre is praised (also as a form of medicine – but where does it fit with the other categories?). No wonder many dieters are confused.

It is time to forget these divisions. Recent attempts to preserve the terminology by subdivisions (into saturated fat and polyunsaturated fat, for example; and simple and complex carbohydrates; not to mention monosaccharides, disaccharides, and polysaccharides) merely create a jungle of jargon. And the classification of foods rich in starch as 'carbohydrate', the confusion of starch with sugar, and the refusal to distinguish whole from processed foods (so that wholewheat bread is bracketed with processed sugar as 'carbohydrate' and is commonly believed to have no more value as food) is a series of mistakes, encouraged by food processors, that have damaged the civilian population of the West in this century more than any war.

The important divisions of food were well known in the West before this century. They are between vegetable and animal food; whole and processed food; and fresh and stale food. We eat animal food for taste, processed food for convenience, but we do not need them. Wholewheat bread, legumes and root vegetables well prepared and eaten fresh and lightly cooked, are rich in starch. But their classification as 'carbohydrates' is arbitrary. The carbohydrate in them supplies energy to the body in a natural way, without causing the disturbances that result from eating sugar. But foods rich in starch are also rich in other nutrients. In different proportions, they also contain protein, fat, fibre, vitamins and minerals.

It is not necessary to be a vegetarian to be healthy. But it is necessary to re-think the relationship between animal and vegetable foods. 'Meat and two veg' is the wrong balance. The chief ingredients in a meal should be cereal or vegetable: so that, for example, the Italian staples of spaghetti and other pastas with olive oil, flavoured in different combinations with vegetables or herbs or cheese or meat, is good food (and better still if the pasta is wholewheat). Meat and dairy produce, now a staple in the West, should merely accompany cereals and vegetables or at the least should be eaten only occasionally. And while animal food eaten sparingly is of course nutritious, processed stale food is inferior to whole fresh food.

All whole grains – wheat, corn, rice, millet, rye, oats – contain protein. So do the legumes – peas, beans, lentils. And so do tubers — potatoes, for example. Many dried beans have as high a protein content as meat; and nuts and seeds are rich in protein and also vegetable fat. We think of meat as protein and therefore as good for us, but much of the meat we eat could almost as well be classified as fat, rather than protein. Even if it has no visible fat, the flesh of meat from animals that are reared in cages and get no exercise, is shot through with fat; and animal fat is certainly implicated in heart disease.

Good food is food that goes bad

On page 144 is a comparison of the nutritive quality of five common foods commonly lumped together as 'carbohydrates': potatoes (fresh, baked in their skins); a whole cereal (wholewheat bread), compared with a processed cereal (white bread); a legume (lentils); and processed sugar.

Unlike fibre, starch is nourishing: it supplies energy to the body and brain. But like fibre, the special quality of starch in its natural form is that it acts as a package for other nutrients – protein, fat, natural sugar, vitamins and minerals. The processing of food means that food can be preserved, and can travel and be stored for long periods of time. But processing is at the expense of nourishment. As a rule of thumb, good food is food that can go bad.

Compare the foods in the table. First, look at the value of the much-despised potato. Potatoes are an important source of vitamin C, especially so when they are new and eaten with their skins. They are a useful source of magnesium and copper. Most importantly, they are a rich source of potassium. Most people in the West consume too much sodium (in the form of salt) and not enough potassium. There is conclusive evidence that excess sodium is a cause of high blood pressure, which in turn increases the risk of heart disease. There is new evidence, summarised

132

in the last couple of years in *The Lancet*, that food rich in potassium can help to counteract the sinister effect of sodium. In this respect potatoes, together with most fresh vegetables and fruit, are a health-promoting food.

Wholewheat bread is rich in no less than thirteen vitamins and minerals. By contrast, white bread has lost the vitamins occurring naturally in whole grain. By law, British millers have been obliged to restore a certain level of synthetic vitamins B_1 (thiamine) and B_3 (niacin), together with iron and calcium, in order to 'fortify' white flour. As the new edition of this book went to press, the British government is proposing to waive this law, on the grounds that British food is so healthy that the people can afford to eat white bread drained of vitamins and minerals.

Like wholewheat bread, and in common with many vegetables and fruits, lentils are an important source of a number of vitamins and minerals, lost in food processing. And, as a legume (one of the bean and pea family) lentils are also valuable as a source of protein – as are cereals.

In utter contrast to the whole foods in the table, processed sugar is empty of nourishment. Processing always drains nourishment from food; processed sugar is unique in having no nutritive value whatsoever. We eat it at our peril.

When nutrition experts say, as they so often do in newspapers and magazines, that we get all the nourishment we need from a 'normal, balanced and varied' combination of foods, they are in one sense correct. But in a more important sense they are misleading. The fact is that, compared with the food eaten at any other time in history, the food we in the West have eaten for the last six generations is uniquely abnormal, unbalanced and artificially varied. The cuisine food based on meat, dairy produce, processed sugar and flour developed by the middle classes in Western Europe in the eighteenth century as one means of boasting of their riches is still considered good food in Great Britain, the USA, France and other Western countries. Cuisine food is a source of sclerotic energy, and has caused the premature death of countless millions of people in the West. In the long view of history, cuisine food is the revenge of the black slaves on their masters and on the descendants of their masters, who gorged themselves on sugar and on the foods loaded with fat and sugar that they purchased with the profits of the slave trade. Nowadays, though, the Western diseases caused by eating processed sugar are, more and more, diseases of poor people in the West, for foods loaded with sugar, once a luxury, are now, together with foods loaded with animal fat, the most available, if not the cheapest, foods.

Fresh food – and fresh air

The table accompanying this chapter, 'The Staff of Life' (see page 139 – 44) is a guide to peasant food – the healthy food that has been the staple food of people throughout history. Principles of healthy food are easily set out.

Cereals, legumes and tubers, rich in starch and fibre and containing protein, fat, vitamins and minerals, are the natural staple foods of mankind. Of all these foods, wholewheat bread is the single most valuable food that is also a natural staple in the West.

Vegetables and fruit, containing starch or sugar and also vitamins and minerals, are a valuable complement to cereals, legumes and tubers, providing that they are eaten whole and fresh, and raw or undercooked.

Vegetable protein and fat are always a better source of nourishment than animal protein and fat, including dairy products. Nuts are a very valuable source of vegetable protein and fat, as are seeds.

Fresh food is always better than processed food. The closer food is to the earth the better. Vegetables are close to the earth; meat further away; meat from animals that eat meat, such as pigs, further away still.

The recommendations made by the McGovern committee in 1977, the James report, and the Royal College of Physicians in 1983 are all giant steps in the right direction. All these reports broadly follow the lines of a multitude of reports issued by expert committees of doctors and scientists since the 1960s, in America, Canada, Australia, New Zealand, various north European countries, and internationally representative bodies such as the World Health Organisation. World-wide, now, there is general agreement that we in the West should eat less fat and should eat a lot less sugar and salt; that we should prefer protein and fat from vegetable sources; and that we should eat plenty of whole, fresh cereal produce, vegetables and fruit. We eat about the right amount of protein, but should eat more from vegetable sources.

But how much less, and how much more? The expert committees have all tried to work out recommendations which could be achieved by entire populations, with the co-operation of government and industry. That is to say, their recommendations are honourable compromises; and many of the committees have had to deal with pressure from government and industry to maintain the status quo, or at least modify our current Western eating habits only marginally.

Peasant communities eat most of their protein and fat contained within the cereal staples that they eat, together with small amounts of lean meat. Any vegetarian in the West is bound to eat more fat, in nuts and seeds if not in dairy produce. Besides, the fats in whole foods are nourishing. So it is not sensible to recommend that we eat only twelve per cent of our calories in the form of fat. An ideal is about twice that amount, or twenty-five per cent, provided that most fat eaten is of vegetable origin (and therefore contains a lot of polyunsaturates).

So the goal, for those of us who are not prepared to wait for government to take an initiative, is to eat rather less fat than recommended by the expert committees; and, at the same time, to eat rather more whole carbohydrate. It is practically impossible to eat too much cereal in whole form, or vegetables, or fruit for that matter; all are filling.

Again, peasant communities cannot be an exact guide to the amount of processed carbohydrate we should eat. But, there again, my own view is that recommendations to cut intake of processed sugar by forty per cent (McGovern) or fifty per cent (Royal College of Physicians) can be misleading, because this can suggest that halving our present intake is an ideal; which it is not. The ideal is to eat no sugar at all: zero. Nor is it sensible to reserve cakes, biscuits and chocolate, say, for the occasional treat: the best policy is to get over the habit of eating sugar, which takes about a month or three, after which food with processed sugar added tastes sickly. Likewise with salt;

135

the best policy is to stop using it in cooking, stop adding it to food, and so become accustomed to the natural taste of food. So any figure for 'processed carbohydrate' in a list of goals, is not an ideal, but merely allows for the fact that it is not really possible completely to avoid it. Ironically, it is often harder to find whole fresh food, especially whole-wheat bread, in the countryside in Britain; most towns have health food shops nowadays, and the Campaign for Real Bread has had something of the success of the Campaign for Real Ale.

Here are the goals I propose, given the conventional division of foods into protein, fat and carbohydrate; but also making the vital division between foods of animal origin (including dairy produce) and foods of vegetable origin (remembering that cereals are an important source of protein and some fat). The current figures for peasant countries, for Western countries, and as recommended by expert committees like the McGovern committee and the Royal College of Physicians (indicated as McG/RCP) are also given:

Goal for healthy food. Energy consumed from different sources (%)

	Peasant %	Western: %	McG/RCP[1] %	Goal %
Vegetable protein	7	4	–	6
Animal protein[2]	4	8	–	6
Total	*11*	*12*	*12*	*12*
Vegetable fat	9	10	–	15
Animal fat[2]	3	30	–	10
Total	*12*	*40*	*30*	*25*
Whole carbohydrate[3]	70	22	43	55
Processed carbo[4]	7	26	15	8
Total	*77*	*48*	*58*	*63*
Total vegetable foods	93	62	75	84
Total animal foods	7	38	25	16

[1] no separate figures given for vegetable and animal.
[2] including dairy produce.
[3] starch mainly; also sugar from fruit etc.
[4] sugar mainly; also starch from white bread etc.

In the Harveian Oration given to the Royal College of

Physicians in London, in October 1982, Sir Richard Doll, having linked obesity, diabetes, and high risk of heart attacks, as diet-related diseases, had this to say:

> Whether the object is to avoid cancer, coronary heart disease, hypertension, diabetes, diverticular disease, duodenal ulcer, or constipation, there is broad agreement among research workers that the type of diet that is least likely to cause disease is one that provides a high proportion of calories in whole grain cereals, vegetables, and fruit; provides most of its animal protein in fish and poultry; limits the intake of fats, and, if oils are to be used gives preference to liquid vegetable oils; includes very few dairy products, eggs, and little refined sugar.

Some cook books have now been written, designed to encourage us to enjoy delicious food which is also healthy: a short list is included in the 'Further Reading' section of this book. Meanwhile, a couple of tips from Dr Denis Burkitt go a long way to help. After recommending breakfasts of wholewheat bread or sugar-free cereal, he goes on to say:

> If I were asked to make one change only in Western diets it would be that we should eat three times as much bread but almost never white. The changes to make in the main meal would be to eat four or five times as much potato and vegetable as meat, and the potatoes should not be peeled, and not cooked or eaten in fat.

Representatives of the food industry who want to see no real change in our eating habits, claim that we need lots of fat, sugar and salt to make our food 'palatable'. Nonsense. Processing food masks the true, delicious taste of whole food. I've never met anyone who switched to wholewheat bread, who then switched back to white bread.

The most obvious sign that our food, in the West, has been drained of nourishment, is the overweight and obesity all around. The worse the food, the fatter people get, in an attempt to get enough nourishment from food. And the increase of obesity in our society, together with diseases of the alimentary tract and of the cardiovascular system, tell us it is time for a change, to good food and plenty of it.

In the first chapter of this book ('Confessions of a Dieter') I quoted a bewildered passage from one of Dr Robert Atkins' diet books in which he says that, if all else fails, a trip to the Mediterranean is recommended. It 'always seems to help with weight reduction. It may be something in the soil.' And I mentioned my month's holiday in Greece, during which I lost eight pounds. Well, there is no cuisine food in Greece. Greek food remains peasant food, and authentic Greek food is the healthiest in Europe. During my long stay I got as close to the guidelines to healthy food outlined above, as I ever had in my life. Dr Atkins' shot in the dark finds a target.

What I also enjoyed in Greece that summer was plenty of fresh air. And for everybody who wants to lose fat while eating plenty of good food, the recipe is: peasant food, and more air.

Table 2. The Staff of Life

Cereals, legumes, tubers, together with other vegetables, fruit, nuts, and seeds, have been the staff of life of all people throughout the world at all times of human history. Meat and dairy products are also enjoyed by hunter-gatherers, pastoralists, and peasants, but only on occasion and as accompaniments to the staple plant and vegetable foods.

In the last 100 – 150 years, machines and money have together created a catastrophic aberration in the West. Rich people have made animal foods a staple; poor people have had to eat processed food. Most people now eat a combination of animal foods and processed foods. These are the prime cause of 'Western diseases' and also of overweight and obesity.

There are no recipes or instructions in this book. Instead, what follows overleaf is a guide to fifty foods available in Britain and America which, if taken as staple foods, and eaten in appropriate combination, are a good approximation to the peasant food that gives health, prevents disease, and, together with exercise, is proof against overweight and obesity.

The first section gives some examples of cereals: wholewheat flour and bread, and also some breakfast cereals. Wholegrain bread made of cereals other than wheat, is also very nutritious. Some commercial muesli is loaded with sugar: only buy sugar-free muesli, or else make up your own.

Every kind of bean is rich in various vitamins and minerals. If you want to keep beans and legumes for a long time, buy them dried, and never canned.

With root vegetables and leaf vegetables, the key is freshness. Stale vegetables lose much of their goodness. Buy fresh from the market, the farm, or from health food shops. The method of cooking is crucial: if you boil vegetables, do so in only a small amount of water, with little or no salt added; and boil lightly. The best method is steaming. Stir-frying the Chinese way, with a wok, is also good.

All fresh vegetables, and fruit, are nutritious; as are nuts and seeds. Note that most nuts are very fatty.

The staff of life
Some common nutritious foods

per 100g	Water %	Protein %	Fat %	Starch %	Sugar %	Dietary Fibre %	Energy cals
Cereals							
Bran, wheat	8.3	14.1	5.5	23.0	3.8	44.0	206
Bread, wholemeal	40.0	8.8	2.7	39.7	2.1	8.5	216
Crispbread, rye	6.4	9.4	2.1	67.4	3.2	11.7	321
Flour, wholemeal	14.0	13.2	2.0	63.5	2.3	9.6	318
Muesli	8.6	13.2	7.5	47.8	3.9	19.0	388
Oatcakes	5.5	10.0	18.3	59.9	3.1	4.0	441
Puffed Wheat	2.5	14.2	1.3	67.0	1.5	15.4	325
Shredded wheat	7.6	10.6	3.0	67.5	0.4	12.3	324
Legumes, etc.							
Beans:							
broad (boiled)	83.7	4.1	0.6	6.5	0.6	4.2	48
haricot (boiled)	69.6	6.6	0.5	15.8	0.8	7.4	93
baked (in tomato sauce)	73.6	5.1	0.5	5.1	5.2	7.3	64
Lentils	72.1	7.6	0.5	16.2	0.8	3.7	99
Peas, fresh	80.0	5.4	0.4	5.9	1.8	5.2	52
Sweetcorn	65.1	4.1	2.3	21.1	1.7	4.7	123
Tomatoes	93.4	0.9	Tr	11.0	9.1	2.3	14
Root vegetables, tubers							
Carrots	91.5	0.6	Tr	0.1	4.2	3.1	19
Onions	96.6	0.6	Tr	0	2.7	1.3	13
Parsnips	83.2	1.3	Tr	10.8	2.7	2.5	56
Potatoes, new (boiled)	78.8	1.6	0.1	17.6	0.7	2.0	76
Potatoes, old (boiled)	80.5	2.1	0.1	19.3	0.4	1.0	87
Potatoes (baked in jackets)	57.5	2.1	0.1	19.8	0.5	2.0	85
Turnips	94.5	0.7	0.3	0	2.3	2.2	14
Leaf vegetables							
Broccoli tops	89.9	1.8	Tr	0.1	1.5	4.1	18
Brussels sprouts	91.5	2.8	Tr	0.1	1.6	2.9	18
Cabbage	95.7	1.3	Tr	Tr	1.1	2.5	9
Lettuce	95.9	1.0	0.4	Tr	1.2	1.5	12
Spinach	85.1	5.1	0.5	0.2	1.2	6.3	30

Cooking method is boiling unless stated. Light boiling, or steaming, is best.

Two vitamins of which the foods in this table are not good sources, are vitamin B_{12} and vitamin D. B_{12} is in various fish; animal livers; and eggs; D is in milk and cod liver oil; also in sunlight.

The presence of sodium in food is not an advantage. We eat too much sodium and not enough potassium.

Good sources of								*Good sources of*								
B1	B2	B3	Fo	Pa	Bi	E		P	Ca	M	I	Z				
B1	B2	B3	B6	Fo	Pa	Bi		S	P	M	Ps	I	Cu	Z	Su	Cl
B6	Fo	Pa	Bi					S	P	M	I	Z				
B1	B2	B3	B6	Fo	Pa	Bi		S	P	M	Ps	I	Cu	Z	Su	Cl
B2	B3	B6	Fo	E				S	P	M	I	Z				
B6	Fo	Pa	Bi	E				S	P	M	I	Z				
Ni	B6	Fo	E					P	M	I	Z					
Ni	B6	Fo	E					P	I	Z						
A	Pa							P	Ps							
								P	Ps	I	Z					
Fo								S	P	Su	Cl					
A	B1	B2						P	M	Ps	I	Cu	Z			
B6																
B6	Fo							S	P	M						
A	Fo	Bi	C	E				P								
A	C															
C								P								
Fo	C	E						P								
B6	C							P	M	Cu						
B6	C							P	M	Cu						
B6	C							P	M	Cu						
Fo								P								
A	B2	B6	C	E				P								
A	B6	C						P								
A	B6	Fo	C					P	Ca							
A	Fo	C						P	Ps							
A	B2	B6	Fo	C	E			P	Ca	M	I					

Key

Vitamins		*Minerals*	
A	Carotene	S	Sodium
B1	Thiamine	P	Potassium
B2	Riboflavin	Ca	Calcium
B3	Niacin	M	Magnesium
B6	Pyridoxine	Ps	Phosphorus
Fo	Folic Acid	I	Iron
Pa	Pantothenic Acid	Cu	Copper
Bi	Biotin	Z	Zinc
C	Ascorbic Acid	Su	Sulphur
E		Cl	Chloride

The staff of life
Some common nutritious foods

per 100g	Water %	Protein %	Fat %	Starch %	Sugar %	Dietary Fibre %	Energy cals
Fruit							
Apples	84.3	0.2	Tr	0.1	9.1	2.0	35
Apricots	86.6	0.6	Tr	0	6.7	2.1	28
Bananas	70.7	1.1	0.3	3.0	16.2	3.4	79
Blackberries	82.0	1.3	Tr	0	6.2	7.3	29
Currants, black	77.4	0.9	Tr	0	6.6	8.7	28
Currants, red	82.8	1.1	Tr	0	4.4	8.2	21
Damsons	77.5	0.5	Tr	0	9.6	4.1	38
Figs, green	84.6	1.3	Tr	0	9.5	2.5	41
Grapes, black	80.7	0.5	Tr	0	13.0	0.3	51
Grapes, white	79.3	0.6	Tr	0	16.1	0.9	63
Lemons	85.2	0.8	Tr	0	3.2	5.2	15
Oranges	86.1	0.8	Tr	0	8.5	2.0	35
Peaches	86.2	0.6	Tr	0	9.1	1.4	37
Prunes (stewed)	60.5	1.3	Tr	0	20.4	8.1	82
Raspberries	83.2	0.9	Tr	0	5.6	7.4	25
Sultanas	18.3	1.8	Tr	0	64.7	7.0	250
Nuts							
Almonds	4.7	16.9	53.5	0	4.3	14.3	567
Brazil nuts	8.5	12.0	61.5	2.4	1.7	9.0	619
Chestnuts	51.7	2.0	2.7	29.6	7.0	6.8	470
Coconut, fresh	42.0	3.2	36.0	0	3.7	13.6	351
Peanuts, fresh	4.5	24.3	49.0	5.5	3.1	8.1	570
Peanut butter	1.1	22.6	53.7	6.4	2.1	7.6	601
Walnuts	23.5	10.6	51.5	1.8	3.2	5.2	525

Two vitamins of which the foods in this table are not good sources, are vitamin B12 and vitamin D. B12 is in various fish; animal livers; and eggs; D is in milk and cod liver oil; also in sunlight.

The presence of sodium in food is not an advantage. We eat too much sodium and not enough potassium.

Table compiled by Kathy Crilley, Chief source of information: *McCance and Widdowson's The Composition of Foods* edited by A A Paul and D A T Southgate (HMSO 1978).

Vitamins — Good sources of	Minerals — Good sources of
A	P
A	P
C E	P M
Bi C E	P
Bi C	P
A B1 Pa C E	S Ca I
B6	P
	P
	P
B6 Pa C	P Ca
Fo C	P
A B3	P
A	P I
Bi C	P
B1 B6 E	P M Ps
B2 B3 B6 Fo E	P Ca M I Z
B1 B6 E	P Ca M Ps I Cu Z Su
B2 B6 Bi	P M
B6 C Fo	S P I
B1 B3 B6 Fo Pa E	P M I Z
B6 Fo Pa E	S P M I Z
B1 B3 Fo Pa E	P Ca M Ps I Z

Key

Vitamins		Minerals	
A	Carotene	S	Sodium
B1	Thiamine	P	Potassium
B2	Riboflavin	Ca	Calcium
B3	Niacin	M	Magnesium
B6	Pyridoxine	Ps	Phosphorus
Fo	Folic Acid	I	Iron
Pa	Pantothenic Acid	Cu	Copper
Bi	Biotin	Z	Zinc
C	Ascorbic Acid	Su	Sulphur
E		Cl	Chloride

Table 3. *The nutritional value of five foods. Percentages are of any given weight. Figures in bold: nutrients of which the food is an important source.*

per 100g		Pota-toes	Bread (whole-wheat)	Bread (white)	Lentils	Sugar (pro-cessed)
Water	%	71.0	40.0	39.0	72.1	tr
Protein	%	2.6	**8.8**	**7.8**	**7.6**	tr
Fat	%	0.1	2.7	1.7	0.5	0
Starch[1]	%	24.4	39.7	47.9	16.2	0
Sugar[1]	%	0.6	2.0	2.0	0.8	**105**[2]
Fibre	%	**2.5**	**8.5**	2.7	3.7	0
Energy	cals	105	216	233	99	394
Vitamins:						
A (Carotene)	µg	tr	0	0	**60.0**	0
Thiamine (B1)	mg	0.1	**0.26**	**0.18**[3]	**0.5**	0
Riboflavin (B2)	mg	0.04	**0.1**	0.03	**0.2**	0
Niacin (B3)	mg	1.2	**3.9**	1.4[3]	2.0	0
Pyridoxine (B6)	mg	**0.2**	0.14	0.04	0.11	0
Cobalamin (B12)	µg	0	0	0	0	0
Folic Acid (B)	µg	10.0	**22.0**	6.0	1.0	0
Pantothenic acid (B)	mg	0.2	**0.6**	0.3	0.3	0
Biotin (B)	µg	tr	**6.0**	1.0	0	0
C (Ascorbic acid)	mg	**30.0**[4]	0	0	tr	0
D	µg	0	0	0	0	0
E	mg	0.1	0.2	tr	0	0
Minerals:						
Sodium	mg	8.0	**540.0**[5]	**540.0**[5]	12.0	tr
Potassium	mg	**680.0**	220.0	100.0	**210.0**	2.0
Calcium	mg	9.0	23.0	**100.0**[3]	13.0	2.0
Magnesium	mg	**29.0**	**93.0**	26.0	**25.0**	tr
Phosphorus	mg	48.0	**230.0**	97.0	**77.0**	tr
Iron	mg	0.8	**2.5**	**1.7**[3]	**2.4**	tr
Copper	mg	**0.2**	**0.3**	0.1	**0.2**	0.02
Zinc	mg	0.3	**2.0**	0.8	**1.0**	0
Sulphur	mg	42.0	**81.0**	**79.0**	39.0	tr
Chloride	mg	94.0	**860.0**	**890.0**	20.0	tr

[1] starch and sugar together are carbohydrate
[2] processed sugar contains what are in effect super-sweet elements
[3] synthetic vitamins and minerals added after being lost in the milling process
[4] when new and eaten with their skins
[5] not valuable at this level. We eat too much sodium and not enough potassium

CHAPTER FIVE

More Air! More Air!

Nothing affects cheerfulness less than wealth and nothing more than health. Let us seek to maintain cheerfulness. Without appropriate daily exercise no one can remain healthy, because satisfactory completion of all living functions requires movement of the parts concerned as well as of the whole. Aristotle was right to say 'life is motion'.

ARTHUR SCHOPENHAUER
Aphorisms on the Wisdom of Life

The narrower and more limited our lives become, the more vitally necessary people will find it to satisfy their longing for freedom in the hazard of their athletic performance.

ROGER BANNISTER
The First Four Minutes

Oxygen: the vital fuel

Wealth, power and fame have their rewards, but most people who live well manage without them. Sooner or later we all find out that the most valuable prize in life is not a rare external object but a common inborn quality: our health.

We in the West have had a negative attitude towards health. We spend the first part of our lives thinking nothing of it, and the second part afraid of losing it. We have been preoccupied not with good health but with ill-health; not with well-being but with disease. An unorthodox but apt definition of 'technology' is 'a means whereby we avoid experiencing our own lives'. Medical technology – the medicine of drugs and surgery where the money, power, newspaper headlines and Nobel Prizes

145

are – discourages us from being responsible for our own health. A long-running BBC Television series has the revealing title *Your Life in Their Hands*. We have the same attitude to doctors and surgeons as the little child who cries out 'Mummy, take the pain away!'

We associate the entire concept of disease with what is in fact a single type of disease: infections, which, while they can largely be prevented by good sanitation, can also be checked or cured by modern medicine. We tend to think of disease as a visitation, as bad luck, as something for which we have no responsibility. We ignore deficiency diseases, caused by lack of nourishment from food, because we assume they do not exist in the West. And we fear the misnamed 'degenerative' diseases of the heart, lungs and blood vessels, and of the gut. In some way we imagine that these, too, are visitations, whereas they are properly named 'Western' diseases, because they are caused by the circumstances in which we live and by our own habits.

It was not always so. The awareness that our good health is our responsibility, a treasure to be protected, is contained in our language. The words 'salute' and 'salutation' derive from *salus*, the Latin word for 'health'. It also means 'safety'. The common French and Italian greetings – *Salut!* and *Salute!* – are wishes for good health and well-being. In this country, greetings are more muted. But on formal occasions, speakers will propose each others' health; and sometimes over drinks, if the occasion seems right, you may toast a friend with the words 'your good health'. The old knowledge is still there, although half-buried.

As with good health, so with the universal element in our environment: air. People who spend most of their time sitting or lying down, especially town and city dwellers, pay no attention to air. After all, as well as being everywhere, it is invisible. Scientists look for new drugs as zealously as alchemists looked for gold. In both cases, the irony is that the most precious element is the most common. Without air we die within five minutes. People who lead active lives value air. But, even more than with good health, people who lead sedentary lives remember the value of air only in extremity. On the point of drowning, the swimmer has one thought in mind; likewise, the person hemmed in by street crowds. The cry is the same. 'More air! More air!'

Oxygen is that part of air which is vital to all the functions of the body. Just as fuel is burned in a flame of oxygen to provide energy in the·form of heat, so oxygen transforms the fuel we eat – food – into all the types of energy that make up life itself; not of course literally in a flame, but by agents in the body that oxidise the food. The dictionary defines 'food' as 'what one takes into the system to maintain life and growth'. This is why the great nutritionist Sir Robert McCarrison wrote: 'Strictly speaking oxygen and water are to be regarded as foods, for of all the supplies on which the cells of the body are dependent they are the chief.'

Which comes first, then: food or oxygen? In one sense the question has no meaning, for we need both, just as a domestic fire has no being without both fuel and oxygen. While the body's fire of course produces no flame, it produces energy in all the forms the body needs. And just as a domestic fire may burn well and brightly with different amounts of fuel and with different draughts, so we can live and thrive at very different levels of energy balance, between the energy supplied by food and that by oxygen.

The desire to be fit

In a vital sense, though, oxygen comes first. The purpose of the new-born infant's first cry is to take air into its lungs. Most people in the West are in a double bind. Not only do they suffer from eating processed, unnatural foods. They also suffer because they do not take the exercise that was a natural part of life before the car was invented. The first move to be free from this bind is to take in more oxygen, by means of appropriate exercise. The issue with food is not quantity, but quality. But the issue with oxygen is one of quantity: almost all of us will thrive if we get more of it. And once we start to use more oxygen, remarkable things start to happen.

In Spring 1982 I launched what became known as the

147

Fun Runner '82 project with *Running* magazine. Having started to jog in 1978, I had run my first marathon, in Paris in 1980, and started to write a column for *Running*. In 1981 I launched the *London 1982/50* project. The title was meant to convey the project's aim: to train fifty men and women for the second London marathon in 1982. The project worked; and so I and about a dozen of the *1982/50* participants decided to encourage a group of absolute beginners to train, not for a marathon, but to complete the *Sunday Times* National Fun Run five months later, in September 1982. This was *Fun Runner '82*.

We reckoned that the Hyde Park Fun Run, which is two and a half miles long, was an attainable goal. 'To qualify, you have to be an absolute beginner,' I wrote.

> I'm looking for people who have never kept fit on any regular basis. I shall be especially interested if you're overweight, or smoke, or have had any history of debilitating illness, or in general feel that you're in such bad shape that the Fun Run seems an Everest.

The applications poured in, from couples, from men, from women.

> We suddenly realised we were getting old and out of condition when we got a dog that needed a lot of exercise.

This was from a couple aged twenty-eight. An ex-smoker who was toying with the idea of becoming an ex-drinker wrote:

> After the excesses of Christmas I looked into the mirror and was horrified to see a flabby 5'11", 14 stone, balding local government officer. Two of these factors could not be reversed, but I decided to do something about my weight and fitness.

Most of the letters were from people who thought, correctly, that they were overweight. One mother said that her family loved swimming, but that she no longer went because she was ashamed of her size. Two other letters from women said:

> I am twenty-eight, and have progressively got less and less fit during the last five years. My energy output is very low as I have an office job that entails sitting down all day. The time has come when I would love to be fit again.

And, from a middle-aged mother:

> Is this the answer to the feeling that my waist is sinking into my hips, is this the self-discipline I have vaguely been feeling I need?

Most of the overweight people were women whose weight had increased to, and then beyond, ten stone and who had discovered that dieting doesn't work. Some had been humiliated by the emphasis on competitive sport at school:

> I was overweight during my school years and pretty useless at sports, always being the one that the coach had to wait for after the cross-country.

Many recalled a lost energy. These letters were wistful, moving, sometimes resigned, a few despairing:

> I have for some time felt generally below par and lacking in energy – the lack of positive health – since I came to London from the countryside.

Eventually I received 130 applications. The first eighty-four were analysed: four were asthma sufferers, three from people with high blood pressure already diagnosed. One person had a heart murmur. Other conditions included a pulmonary embolism (recovered); slipped discs (two), back problems, bronchitis, hernia, curvature of the spine and epilepsy. One of the most touching letters said:

> Medically the last eighteen months have been rotten. Head, leg and shoulder injuries and an unknown virus took it out of me spiritually as well as physically. However, I feel much better now, except that I feel the strain of being very overweight.

149

Of the eighty-four, twenty-two smoked, twenty-three had given up; forty-nine were definitely overweight; thirty-eight had taken no exercise since school and forty said they had exercised 'a bit'. Their ages ranged from eighteen to fifty-five; most people were in their thirties and forties. The average age was early to mid thirties.

Eventually sixty-four people were chosen to take part in *Fun Runner '82*. The fittest participant was, at fifty-five, the oldest: John Routledge, a company director. The previous summer he had been given an executive check-up. He was a bit alarmed at his blood pressure, but was told that it was not unusual for his age. A couple of months later he had a massive heart attack and then clinically 'died'. Afterwards, in hospital, he remembered a conversation with a friend playing snooker; he had leaned over the table to play a ball and couldn't reach. 'Your undercarriage is in the way, John,' said his friend. Out of hospital John started to jog and eat fresh food. He had lost about thirty pounds and was doing five-mile runs when I met him. His experience as a runner should have disqualified him from joining the project; but his experience of heart disease and his subsequent decision to save his own life would, I thought, be valuable.

Vic Burrowes, one of the applicants, had written:

> If I am selected for your programme it could change my whole way of life. You said it might seem an Everest to some people. At the moment I would liken it to climbing the whole Himalayan range.

I was interested to see what would happen to Vic.

The participants in the project all agreed to undertake a series of tests during the five-month training programme, leading up to the goal of the *Sunday Times* National Fun Run. The physiological tests, based on the work of Professor Per-Olof Åstrand in Stockholm, were supervised by Ted Charlesworth and Kevin Sykes of the Human Performance Laboratory at Chester College and had already been used to test the fitness of the Cheshire fire service and police. They were carried out three times: at the start of the project, at the mid-point and at the end of the twenty-one weeks.

As well as measurements of height, weight and various parts of the body, the tests were of blood pressure; body fat percentage (non-essential fat); lung capacity; heart rate; cardiorespiratory fitness (fitness of the heart and lungs); and, finally, 'fitness category'. Everybody wanted to know 'How fit am I?' Fitness category was determined by measuring the fitness of the heart and lungs in terms of the body's capacity to use oxygen, and resulted in the following grades: 'excellent', 'good', 'average', 'below average', and – rock bottom – 'poor'. This grading was based on measurements of tens of thousands of people carried out in Dallas, Texas, by Dr Kenneth Cooper, founder of the Aerobics Institute.

I was also interested to know how far individuals' mood, attitudes and personality might change as a result of exercise and getting fit. So Dr Barrie Gunter, a research psychologist with special knowledge of sport, asked everyone to fill in a long questionnaire at the beginning and end of the project. This was the 'Cattell 16 Personality Factor' test, a standard method of measuring shifts in personality.

I myself devised a questionnaire for everyone to fill in at the mid-point of the project. This was designed to find out why people had joined *Fun Runner '82*; what they were getting out of it; and whether their eating and sleeping habits were changing. I also wanted to find out if people's moods changed as a result of exercise.

How to save the NHS a billion pounds a year

The physiological tests are usually called 'fitness tests'. I prefer the name 'health tests', for what they measure is the health and strength of the heart, lungs and blood vessels. They are not a health check of the whole body, but nonetheless they are important.

It seemed to me at the time, and with more force now, that tests of the sort supervised by Ted Charlesworth and Kevin Sykes, which take about twenty-five minutes to carry out and are suitable for all able-bodied people whatever their level of fitness, should be available as part of a general practitioner's routine examination, not just for private patients but as part of the National Health Service. The machinery is not expensive.

In 1981, 173,649 men and women died of coronary heart disease in Britain. A further 84,738 people died of strokes and hypertensive disease. In the last fifteen years the rate of deaths from heart disease in America has dropped by over twenty-five per cent; Americans are moving towards a healthy diet and are taking more exercise. Translated into British terms the American success would result in over 40,000 lives being saved every year from heart disease alone. But in Britain these lives are not being saved; the rate of death from heart disease has not changed significantly in the last twenty years. Leading British heart disease specialists such as Professor Barry Lewis, Dr Richard Turner, Dr Keith Ball and Professor Geoffrey Rose believe that between thirty and ninety per cent of deaths from heart disease are preventable, by eating healthy food and also by exercise, together with giving up smoking.

William Laing, a leading health economist, states that the total number of working days lost in 1981 in Britain from heart disease was well over twenty-six million, with a further figure of sixteen million working days lost because of strokes and hypertensive disease. In a feature in *The Sunday Times* in July 1983 Laing estimated that if Western diseases in Britain, of which heart disease is the chief, were prevented to the extent they can be prevented, the cost savings to the National Health Service would be over a billion pounds a year – between £881 and £1,541 million, according to different estimates, not counting cancer. We still live in a world, though, where prevention, though cheaper than treatment, is less glamorous, even when the immensely expensive treatment involving coronary by-pass, heart transplants or plastic hearts is unlikely to be effective.

The initial series of physiological tests showed that on average the Fun Runners were a bit overweight and over-fat; that their blood pressure was noticeably above the 'ideal' of 120/80 for women (at 127/91) and somewhat higher for men (at 137/93); and that fitness level was about 'average' for men and a bit 'below average' for women. 'Average' fitness is nothing to be satisfied about; it is what it says, the average for a basically sedentary population.

The averages concealed a wide range of fitness. Of the twenty-five men assessed before they started to exercise, six were 'below average' and two 'poor'. The women's fitness level was lower; of the thirty-two women measured, five were 'below average' and ten 'poor'. The 'poor' rating means you are liable to get out of breath running a bath.

The Fun Runners were formed into six teams, ideally each of ten to a dozen people. Experience shows that this is a good number for a team and allows for a few people to be away (on summer holiday, for instance). Each team had two trainers: these were mostly people from the now-completed *London 1982/50* project who had told me that they had gained so much from their nine months that they wanted to put back some of their enthusiasm, time and experience to the beginner Fun Runners.

Once a week every team met with their trainers. Once a month everybody came together on a Saturday morning in Hyde Park for a 'family' run. Special T-shirts were printed. Everybody was asked to exercise four times a week, preferably evenly spaced, and to keep a diary in which they recorded the times and distances they covered.

When starting an exercise programme, it is crucial to take it easy at first and then build up slowly. At first everybody was asked to jog and walk just over a mile, stopping whenever they liked. (Unfit people can usually run 200 to 400 yards without stopping.) As time went on everybody was encouraged to jog, and then run, further and faster, in their own time and at their own speed. The secret with this kind of training is to take your pulse rate and check to see that it is neither too high nor too low. (A guide to a training programme that able-bodied people can use is in the table 'Health Through Fitness', on pp. 191 – 4.)

At the mid-point of the project everybody had their second fitness tests. Allan Appleton, a forty-six-year-old company director, who had started the project with 'below average' fitness, had risen to 'excellent'. In five months he was to lose twenty-two pounds in weight and thirty per cent of his non-essential body fat. But for him the main benefits at the half-way stage were:

Many, and much appreciated: a tremendous increase in fitness and well-being, the previously unknown pleasure of running

153

with members of my family. I will, for the rest of my life, run and exercise regularly.

You don't often hear people being this enthusiastic about a diet regime. Allan's loss of weight and non-essential fat was unusually high. I spent most time during the project with the 'Inner' team in central London, one of the six teams which included John Routledge and Vic Burrowes. At the half-way stage, after eleven weeks, their results were:

		Body Weight (st:lb)		Body Fat (%)		Fitness category	
	Age	before	after	before	after	before	after
Cinnia Bermingham	36	9:1	8:9	16	14	5	2
Victor Burrowes	46	12:10	11:1	18	14	3	2
Tim Burton	31	11:7	11:11	15	14	4	3
David Dyke	34	10:5	10:0	19	15	4	1
Nick Gray	25	12:1	11:13	13	12	3	1
Lynette Hadfield	39	10:9	10:7	30	27	5	4
Jane Heywood	33	10:6	9:13	13	11	1	1
Teresa Malinowska	27	11:5	11:3	20	14	4	3
Liz Parry	29	11:0	10:11	22	20	5	3
John Routledge	55	11:11	11:9	11	10	2	2
Eileen Ward	27	15:1	15:5	40	38	5	4

Victor Burrowes had lost twenty-three pounds in eleven weeks. He had a sad tale to tell:

> One of the reasons for taking up *Fun Runner '82* was excessive weight. Now, 11 weeks into the project I have lost almost two stone and my clothes still don't fit me! I shall have to buy a new wardrobe.

What's more, Vic swore that he had not been on a diet. Answering my questionnaire about food, he said that, while he was eating less sweets, he was eating more meat, fish, protein, fruit and vegetables. He also turned out to have a natural talent for running: he entered a three-mile race and came second in the forty-six to fifty age category. And he continued to enjoy his beer.

Tim Burton was the fourteen-stone local government officer who had written to me a few months before. Before starting to exercise he had gone on a semi-starvation diet, which he stopped as soon as he started to

154

run. But having dieted he was weakened, and his fitness level at the start was the lowest of all the men. After eleven weeks he had gained over four pounds, but had lost fat.

The most striking example of the way exercise affects body composition rather than weight was Teresa Malinowska, a tall young woman. She had lost a couple of pounds, and was to lose a total of five by the end of five months; but in eleven weeks she lost thirty per cent of her non-essential body fat. Her body shape changed remarkably; as well as looking radiant, from being a bit plump she changed to being lean.

Jane Heywood started – and ended – the fittest in the group. She was in the habit of cycling to work. Eileen Ward was one of the three very over-fat women in the group of sixty-four, none of whom lost weight during the five months of the project, although all lost a small amount of fat. John Routledge showed no change in weight, body fat, or fitness, which was no surprise, because he was not taking any more exercise. At the beginning of the project his blood pressure, now much lower than the year before, was 144/86. In eleven weeks it came down to 120/80: the blood pressure of a young man.

How to prolong your own life

While the project was running I heard a doctor say on BBC radio, without a doubt in his voice, that people with high blood pressure usually had to take drugs indefinitely to reduce the pressure. A leaflet put out by the Flora margarine project for heart disease prevention, found in many health centres, advocates losing weight, eating less salt, and cutting down saturated fats, together with giving up smoking and avoiding tension, as means to reduce blood pressure. No mention of exercise.

Yet in eleven weeks the blood pressure of all those participants who were measured twice fell as follows:

	before	after
Men	137/93	127/82
Women	127/91	121/82

Dr Eoin O'Brien and Professor Kevin O'Malley explain the

significance of these figures in their book *High Blood Pressure*. They take the example of a man somewhat older than most men in *Fun Runner '82*:

A 45 year old man with a systolic pressure of 120 and a diastolic level of 80 may expect to live to over 70 years of age. A man of much the same age with a systolic pressure of 140 and a diastolic of 95 may expect to live six years less.

The fifteen people of the sixty-four who started the five-month project with high blood pressure ended with lower blood pressure. Here is the entire list:

		before	after
Women:	age 36	137/95	108/72
	29	134/105	112/80
	29	134/97	113/69
	39	154/111	135/88
	38	132/114	125/81
	29	136/91	117/79
	47	139/98	130/70
	33	138/81	125/75
Men:	age 46	152/106	130/74
	31	146/91	140/86
	53	158/108	130/90
	25	142/90	135/78
	55	144/86	120/80
	48	140/90	125/66
	26	140/80	122/63

In five months half a dozen people in their late thirties, forties or fifties improved their life expectancy by six years. The man of forty-eight whose blood pressure dropped so remarkably was Rodney Lewis, a north London taxi-driver. Before the project, he said, he was always pushing his window down and shouting and screaming at silly drivers. His new blood pressure brought a new personality with it; he lost his jagged edges and became a calmer man. Vic Burrowes' blood pressure dropped more than twenty points.

Between May and September about ten people dropped out of the project; holidays and other reasons meant that others were not tested three times. Of those who completed the course (and the Fun Run) and were also tested in May, July and September, the men, on average, lost nine pounds of body weight and, more significantly, over twenty per cent of their non-essential body fat. One man, Tim Burton, gained weight in the five months – all lean tissue. One stayed the same; two kept the same weight but lost fat; the rest lost weight and fat.

The women's results were less striking. On average they lost four and a half pounds of weight and ten per cent of their non-essential fat. The three very over-fat women got fitter and completed the two and a half mile Fun Run to tumultuous cheers; but one did not change her weight or shape much, and the other two actually gained weight, while at the same time losing fat, over the five months. Paradoxically, they were the two who, at fourteen stone four and fifteen stone one, had most to lose; both were also short in stature. Leaving these three women aside, the rest, half of whom were overweight, half average or slim, lost about six pounds in five months.

Losing weight was not, it should be said, a principal reason why people joined the project. In July, half-way through, I asked everybody why they had joined, and the most frequently mentioned reasons were 'getting fit', 'feeling good' and 'getting in shape'. Defined in this way, the project was a great success for almost everybody who completed it. This table compares the cardiorespiratory fitness of the thirty-four people who completed all the tests, before and after the project.

| | Men | | Women | |
	before	after	before	after
Excellent	1	11	2	6
Good	2	3	4	8
Average	7	0	1	4
Below average	4	0	5	1
Poor	0	0	8	1

What impressed me equally were the comments people made about their eating habits. In July, half-way through, I asked participants how much they were eating, and if they had changed their food habits in any way. Everyone had been strongly advised to keep their strength up and not diet, and in July only one person said she was on a diet. If anything, people seemed to be eating more, not less.

I also asked if people were spontaneously eating more or less of different types of food. The only outside influence was Audrey Eyton's *F-Plan Diet*, advocating fibre, which became the thing to eat in the summer of 1982. Members of the project were asked to list the types of food they were eating more, or less, of:

Foods	more	less
Meat/fish	10	6
Dairy products	9	10
Sugar/sweets/chocolate	7	18
Cereals and pastas	12	7
Fibre	15	1
Alcohol	10	17
Protein	9	3
Fat	0	14
Carbohydrate	9	6
Vitamins	11	2
Fruit	21	2

The men and the women responded similarly. Replies to questionnaires of this sort must be treated with some caution. Everybody knows that it is a good thing to eat fruit and vegetables, and a bad thing to eat fat, and people no doubt tend to report what they know they ought to do rather than what they actually do. Given this, it was quite striking that ten people said they were drinking more alcohol (usually in the form of beer after runs, judging by the jovial occasions I attended).

The switch away from sugar, sweets and chocolate in favour of cereals and pastas was therefore especially interesting. Sugar and products heavy in sugar are advertised as sources of quick energy, and runners are often (wrongly) told to eat them after a run. By contrast cereals and pastas have a stodgy image, and people who want to lose weight are often (wrongly) told to avoid them. But the Fun Runners moved away from processed foods – sugar, and also products heavy in sugar and fat – and moved towards whole foods.

After eleven weeks of their exercise programme, the Fun Runners were approximating to the recommendations of the Royal College of Physicians spontaneously, without any prompting from doctors, books, trainers, or from me.

The implications of these results are exciting. They suggest that when people become active their bodies tend to adapt, to prefer foods rich in nourishment that supply energy at a natural rate and to avoid foods poor in nourishment that supply energy at an unnaturally fast rate. To put it another way, the fit body becomes healthy partly by adapting to prefer healthy food. Moreover, one vitamin, thiamine (B_1) is used particularly in activity; and many whole starchy foods are rich in thiamine.

I mentioned these findings to a leading expert on diabetes; for it is now recognised that adult-onset diabetes can be treated by cutting out sugar and by eating whole food rich in starch and fibre. 'Ah,' he said. 'You're one of those people who believes in the wisdom of the body.' Yes, I said, I supposed that I was.

On 26 September the members of the project had the time of their lives, running in the *Sunday Times* National Fun Run. A lot of the men had become pretty fast: most of them completed the two and a half mile course in under eighteen minutes, and Rodney Lewis beat me by a second (he was in the same race as me, but I never managed to catch him). The women were less competitive. Debbie Hoyle, a young mother of two children, finished in eighteen minutes twenty-six seconds; and Cinnia Bermingham, who had written to me five months before saying that she got out of breath running for a bus, finished in nineteen minutes and six seconds. The biggest cheers were for the women in their late thirties and forties, some of whom had developed a fair turn of speed.

After five months, the project had encouraged a lot of people to become fit. But very much more had happened, besides. People had lost weight, lost body fat and changed shape. Their blood pressure had come down to that of young people, and, correspondingly, their ability to use oxygen had increased dramatically. They had proved to their own satisfaction that runners are healthy people.

Dr Barrie Gunter made his own assessment of the project. He said that after twenty-one weeks of exercise the Fun Runners were more self-confident and emotionally stable, more self-assured, more relaxed and composed. He was especially interested in how friendly most people had become. He said:

> My feeling is that this is partly a result of taking part in a group
> activity with other people all striving towards the same goal;
> as well as training their bodies, people were also exercising
> their skills in dealing with other people. The less fit had been
> helped and encouraged by the more fit.

These benefits are part of what running is all about.
Running is, almost uniquely, a social activity, because you
can not only run with companions (as opposed to
competing against an opponent) but also talk with your
companions all the time you are running – well, at least
until the run becomes a little competitive.

Bill East was fifty-three. At the end of the project his
blood pressure had dropped by more than twenty points.
He said:

> I have achieved far more than I thought possible. I can run 4½
> miles non-stop, my weight, blood pressure and resting heart-
> rate are all down, and without trying my smoking is down.
> And I have learned that the body does not deteriorate pro rata
> with age: I am not that far behind youngsters half my age.

I was surprised to discover Bill's age. He looks ten years
younger. Will Chapman was one of the leaders of the *Fun
Runner* project. In 1971, weighing sixteen and a half
stone, he had a heart attack. Afterwards, like John
Routledge, he started jogging and became a marathon
runner. He said:

> Non-runners ask me what I get out of pounding the streets. My
> weight is a normal 12½ stone and yet I eat and drink what I
> want; I'm told I look young for my 45 years and I feel great.

Will was a member of the previous *London 1982/50*
project, but there is no need to run marathons to benefit
from exercise. Bobbie Randall was forty-seven and the
mother of six. 'I'm the only fatty left in the family,' she
explained, writing to join *Fun Runner '82*. 'My job is
sedentary, as are my hobbies. I just cannot shift my
surplus. Perhaps it's been around too long.' In five months

she lost eleven pounds, her blood pressure was down from 139/98 to 130/70, her ability to use oxygen had almost doubled, and she ran the Fun Run in twenty-three minutes fifty seconds, coming seventy-first out of 141 in her age category. In January 1983 she won a handicap race of over four miles organised by the Serpentine Running Club. Rodney Lewis had been a previous winner of this race.

Lose weight: eat more

I was already aware that Professor Peter Wood was mounting similar projects in California with a number of colleagues. Wood, an Englishman who has lived in the USA for twenty years, is deputy director of the Heart Disease Prevention Unit at Stanford University, and a veteran of over seventy marathon races. He is also jointly responsible for a nation-wide club of veteran joggers and runners, the '50 + Association'.

In 1976 he mounted a seventeen-week exercise programme for twenty-two very overweight women aged between thirty and fifty-two. Most had previously tried and failed to lose weight by dieting. The women also attended classes designed to encourage awareness of their eating habits, but were not told to diet. In practice, most of them made moderate reductions in the amount of food they ate.

At the end of the programme, average weight had fallen by nine pounds. Body fat had decreased by eleven pounds, while lean tissue had increased by two pounds. Resting heart rate and heart rate recovery after exercise also decreased, as did blood pressure. Wood's professional speciality is the study of blood lipids; that is to say, fat in the blood.

It is now known that the volume of fat in the blood does not necessarily itself indicate a high risk of heart disease. What matters is the type of fat. It is 'low density lipoprotein' (LDL), large, sticky globules of fat bound up with protein, that is linked with heart disease. LDL increases when large amounts of processed sugar are eaten, and in time the sticky globules line and clog the

161

blood vessels. 'High density lipoprotein' (HDL) by contrast, small, smooth globules of fat and protein, is not only harmless but may in effect scour the blood vessels, renewing them and making them healthier.

Wood found that exercise increased the volume of HDL and decreased that of LDL, and also significantly increased the proportion of HDL to LDL. His findings have been confirmed by work done by Dr Peter Williams of BUPA, in London.

Wood's next projects were more ambitious. He compared the amount of food eaten by thirty-four male and twenty-seven female runners aged between thirty-five and fifty-nine, and averaging thirty-five to forty miles a week.

As might be expected, the runners were considerably leaner and lighter than a sedentary 'control' group. But the runners were eating more – a lot more.

Male runners consumed 2959 calories a day, vs 2361 for controls. The corresponding mean values for female runners and controls were 2386 and 1871 calories a day, respectively.

The runners were considerably lighter than the non-runners. The male runners were eating almost half as much again per pound of body weight as male non-runners; women more than half as much again. Lose weight: eat more. Gain weight: eat less. As the Royal College of Physicians' report on obesity said in 1983:

The role of physical activity in the development of increased adiposity may well have been under-emphasised . . . There will need to be an appreciable and permanent change in society's attitude to exercise.

Not everybody wants to run thirty-five to forty miles a week. And sedentary people often assume that the only way to lose weight and fat and become slim by running is either to have run all your life or else to run great distances. Another study by Peter Wood, of middle-aged women who played ten hours of tennis a week, compared with a control group of sedentary women who on average weighed over 16 pounds more, disproves that. Wood: 'We found that the tennis players' food intake was 2417 calories a day, while the overweight women ate only 1490. That's an enormous difference.'

That is not to say that the runners and the tennis players studied were eating a great deal: but at 2400 to 3000 calories a day their energy intake was sufficient to ensure them enough nourishment from vitamins and minerals, given that the food eaten was nutritious. Rather, it was the inactive people who ate little; in the tennis study, the inactive women, who on average were overweight, consumed no more energy than many diet books recommend for a semi-starvation regime.

The full significance of this pioneering work becomes clear when the energy value of running and playing tennis is measured. Running uses about nine to twelve calories a minute more than sitting, playing tennis about five calories more. Hence the estimate made by Dr John Garrow that running a marathon consumes about 2500 calories. Hence, also, the notion that you have to walk up and down Ben Nevis to work off the effects of a hearty meal.

The runners studied by Wood were eating 550 calories a day more than the non-runners. According to the usual calculations, in order to run that extra energy off, at a brisk seven to eight miles an hour, they would have to run for about an hour every day, or fifty to sixty-five miles a week – far more than they were actually running. Even a fast runner would have to do forty-five miles a week to burn off 600 calories a day. Moreover, the runners were lighter than the non-runners.

The same calculation applied to the tennis players has even more remarkable results. According to the books, you would have to play tennis for 200 minutes a day to burn off 1000 calories, which is twenty-three hours twenty minutes every week. In fact, the tennis-players were playing less than half that time. Something is missing from the calculations.

Exercise speeds you up

In theory, according to the books, exercise is not a particularly effective way of losing weight and fat. In practice, according to experience, exercise is a most effective way of losing some weight and more fat. Moreover, in Peter Wood's words:

> It is a fallacy that thinner, active people eat less than overweight sedentary people. In fact, they eat more. We have proved that food intake increases among those who exercise and decreases among the sedentary.

Just as dieting slows you down, exercise of the right type speeds you up. Books recommending exercise usually give charts showing the energy value of different forms of physical activity. But the measurements on which these charts are based, while being accurate as far as they go, do not allow for the fact that certain types of exercise, sustained at a steady intensity for relatively long periods of time, speed up the metabolic rate, not only while you are exercising, but also afterwards.

As long ago as 1935 it was calculated that vigorous and sustained exercise raises the metabolic rate. This early study estimated that resting metabolic rate could be raised by exercise by as much as twenty-five per cent for fifteen hours afterwards, and by perhaps ten per cent for forty-eight hours afterwards.

The resting metabolic rate of a sedentary woman of average weight has been estimated to account for around 1250 calories a day. In round terms this is one calorie a minute, or sixty calories an hour. Using the figures quoted above, the right kind of exercise, for such a woman, could therefore be worth an extra fifteen calories an hour for fifteen hours (equals 225 calories); and an extra six calories an hour for forty-eight hours (equals 288 calories). Therefore, in round figures, the true energy value of such exercise could be around 500 calories in addition to the energy used during the exercise.

And this, of course, is why the relatively lean women tennis players studied by Professor Wood were eating almost twice as much food as the sedentary – and relatively fat – women.

Any physiologist knows that the metabolic effect of vigorous exercise continues after the exercise has finished. In scientific language, exercise that puts an unusual load on muscles stresses the muscles and breaks

164

down muscle fibre (this process is termed 'catabolism'). Thereafter, the muscle fibre is built up again ('anabolism') to become stronger and more able to withstand exercise. This 'training effect' enables anybody to become fitter, simply by means of repeated exercise. The metabolic cycle, of catabolism and anabolism (muscle break-down and build-up) of course does not all happen during the exercise; and of course, it requires energy. The only question is – how much energy?

Active people know that exercise affects the body after the exercise has finished, as a matter of everyday observation. Stiff muscles, the day after hard exercise, need more time to continue building up. A very common mistake made by people eager to improve their fitness, is to exercise daily, on stiff muscles, which then break down further and become injured beyond immediate repair. Anyone not an athlete should not, in my view, train hard more than four times a week, for this reason.

Also, people who progress from being sedentary to being active enjoy the experience of feeling warmer all the time. What this means, in scientific language, is that their metabolic rate is higher – all the time. Extra body heat is being generated, day and night, by exercise.

In 1976 The Sports Council of England and Wales commissioned Professor Peter Fentem, a leading British sports physiologist, to prepare a study, 'The Case For Exercise'. After three years of investigation, one of Dr Fentem's conclusions was:

> Exercise has a stimulating effect on metabolism which persists throughout the day, raises the metabolic rate and leads to the loss of appreciably more fat than would have been predicted for the exercise undertaken.

This statement refers to the fact that vigorous exercise, when sustained over a period of time, has a doubly beneficial effect on the metabolic rate. In a previous chapter ('Dieting Makes You Fat') it was shown that a lean person may require 300 calories a day more than a fat person of the same weight, simply because of being lean. And this is a major reason why dieting is futile, because it has the accumulative effect of replacing lean tissue with body fat. Since lean tissue is much more metabolically

165

active than body fat, the result is that the dieter's metabolism slows down.

Exercise, when vigorous and sustained, has the opposite effect. Metabolic rate is a function of lean body mass: the more lean tissue people have, the higher their metabolic rate, other things being equal. Exercise has the effect of using body fat as fuel, and at the same time building up lean tissue. The fitter you are, the more you can, and should, eat.

The facts that metabolism is dynamic, and that exercise using a lot of oxygen speeds up the metabolic rate, are so important and basic that people, once again, often say to me: 'If all this is true, why haven't I heard it before?'

Fit and healthy people tend to be able to do without junk food and drugs; and junk food and drugs are very profitable commodities. That's one, cynical, reason. And preventive medicine remains the Cinderella of the medical profession, although that is now beginning to change. But there are a number of practical reasons why what is written here is likely to be news to many readers.

The procedure involved in measuring metabolic rate is complicated and laborious. Far more measurements have been made of changes in metabolic rate as a result of dieting, fasting and over-eating than as a result of exercise, simply because it is easier to measure people sitting down than to measure them running over a period of months.

Diet books and studies of obesity pay little attention to the role of oxygen because until recently the only group of people, mountaineers and divers aside, with a direct interest in the relationship of oxygen and energy balance were athletes. Exercise physiology, the science concerned with the effects of oxygen on the human body, was a specialised department, of general interest only to physical education teachers and trainers. Ordinary people took oxygen for granted, just as nutritionists who measure the energy content of food by burning it in a 'calorimeter' take it for granted.

But now the explosion of interest in exercise among ordinary citizens, and in particular the enthusiasm for jogging and running, is turning hundreds of thousands of previously fat people into athletes. These people find they no longer need to diet, and become interested in eating lots of good food instead. The scientists who study energy balance in fat people and those who study energy balance in fit people are beginning to get together.

The research now being done on exercise and metabolic rate is almost all new, and would have been hard to mount until recently for another practical reason. Research needs subjects. Until the late 1970s virtually everybody in Western countries remained sedentary throughout life, or else was active only when young. A few people remained active throughout life. For practical purposes it was unknown for people to get more active as they got older. Professor J N Morris, whose studies of London bus conductors and drivers in the 1950s showed that, because they walked up and down the stairs of the double-decker buses, conductors were less likely to suffer heart disease, did his work at a time when doctors commonly believed that exercise was bad for you.

Conclusive studies of the effects of exercise on metabolism can only be carried out on people who, like the sixty-four Fun Runners, have decided for themselves to progress from being *homo sedentarius to homo sportivus.*

What is the effect of long-term, regular exercise on metabolic rate, on the quantity and quality of food eaten, on weight, shape, fitness and health? How much exercise is needed to become fit and healthy? Are some forms of exercise better than others? How long should exercise sessions take, and how regular should they be? The Royal College of Physicians' 1983 report on obesity says:

The physiological effects of short periods of moderately intensive exercise are well defined, and a minimum of 20 minutes of moderate activity three times a week seems sufficient to maintain cardio-vascular responses to physical activity. This degree of activity also seems to play an important role in improving an individual's sense of well-being.

That is to say, a certain type of exercise, carried out with a certain regularity for a certain amount of time, makes you feel good, makes you fit, and makes you healthy. The exercise that produces these effects is now known as 'aerobic' exercise.

The types of exercise

Dr Kenneth Cooper is the founding father of the aerobic movement, first in the USA, and now throughout the world. In his book *Aerobics* he divides exercise into four types.

Isometrics tense the muscles against themselves or against an immovable object. Isometric exercises strengthen skeletal muscle and are useful for the bedridden and for astronauts. Sometimes they are recommended for executives and office workers who want to do battle with their desks.

Isotonics contract the muscles and also involve movement. As well as strengthening muscle they can make the body more supple or bulkier with muscle. They promote well-being as well as muscular fitness. Examples are the Canadian Air Force exercises in the popular book *Physical Fitness*, weight training, school PT and yoga.

Anaerobic exercise itself divides into two types: either too easy, or too hard, to be aerobic. Literally, 'aerobic' means 'with oxygen'; and students of exercise have until recently been accustomed to refer to any activity as 'aerobic' simply because it uses air. Now, though, the term 'aerobic' has come to refer to exercise that makes a sustained demand on the heart and lungs and which uses the big muscles of the body, such as the muscles of the legs.

Anaerobic exercise may be so gentle, or so brief, that it makes no real demands on the heart and the lungs. Alternatively, anaerobic exercise may be so intense that after a short while it cannot be sustained; the body cannot supply the volume of oxygen required and goes into 'oxygen debt', signalled by severe breathlessness.

Aerobic exercise occupies the middle ground between the two types of anaerobic exercise. It is neither gentle nor intense. It is exercise sustained at a steady, vigorous level for a considerable period of time.

Isometrics and isotonics do not increase the amount of oxygen used by the body, unless they are accompanied by systematic and sustained breathing exercises. Thus, they do not strengthen the heart, lungs and blood vessels and so improve fitness as distinct from health.

Any kind of sprinting, whether running, cycling or swimming, is by this definition anaerobic, for sprinting cannot be sustained for more than a couple of minutes. 'Aerobics', now popular in Great Britain and the USA, is a mixture of dance and exercise which is aerobic simply because, properly taught, it is sustained for over five minutes at a time. What constitutes aerobic activity depends on the state of fitness and health of the individual. A gentle jog may be anaerobic for the fit young person because it is too easy; for the unfit middle-aged person it may be anaerobic because it is too hard.

Dr Cooper defines aerobic exercise for young people as follows:

> If the exercise is vigorous enough to produce a sustained heart rate of 150 beats a minute or more, the training-effect benefits begin about five minutes after the exercise starts and continue as long as the exercise is performed. If the exercise is not vigorous enough to produce or sustain a heart rate of 150 beats a minute, but is still demanding oxygen, the exercise must be continued considerably longer than five minutes, the total period of time depending on oxygen consumed.

Fitness training may develop physical speed, strength or endurance in different proportions, depending on its purpose. This is true for the Olympic athlete, the patient recovering from a heart attack and for ordinary citizens, whatever their initial level of fitness.

The athlete trains in order to improve performance. A sprinter develops speed rather than endurance; a marathon runner develops endurance rather than strength. Training for many sports is specialist. And people may or may not be healthy, depending on the type of training they undertake. Exercise that develops strength or speed but not endurance is anaerobic. Exercise that develops endurance is aerobic, because endurance is achieved by training the body's capacity to use oxygen. Aerobic exercise promotes health through fitness because, by its sustained use of oxygen, it strengthens the heart, lungs, blood vessels and other vital organs, as well as the muscles.

This is why, as Dr Cooper states, in order to be aerobic exercise must elevate the heart rate past a certain point for a certain period of time. The reason why sprinting is anaerobic is because it uses oxygen stored within the muscle itself, which is soon exhausted. On the other hand jogging (at a speed appropriate to the physical condition of the individual) is aerobic, because it uses oxygen breathed in from the air.

What is 'aerobic' exercise?

The key to aerobic exercise is that it should be sustained for five minutes at the very least, preferably for ten minutes; and that during this time the heart rate should be elevated to sixty to eighty per cent of its maximum. This duration and intensity has been determined by doctors and scientists specialising in the heart and in exercise physiology. Below the level of sixty per cent, exercise will not have an aerobic effect; that is to say, it will not strengthen the cardiovascular system. And only very fit people can gain aerobic benefit from exercise above the eighty per cent level.

Some men (it's almost always men) push themselves too hard on exercise programmes, and there is even a condition known as 'positive addiction': the jogger cannot do without the daily session. I see nothing but good in running a lot if you enjoy it; but I always advise people, including runners training for marathons, to run no more than four days a week.

Progress in running and other aerobic activities is much like progress in any other area of life: it goes by fits and starts. You reach a certain level, then stick on this 'plateau' for a while, sometimes quite a long time; then there is a 'breakthrough' to a higher level. It's important not to expect progress to be steady. Many training programmes make that mistake.

Here are the most common questions people ask me

about aerobic exercise. First: which sports and activities are aerobic and which are anaerobic? Second: how can I discover when my heart rate is elevated to sixty to eighty per cent of maximum? Third: how long should I exercise each day and each week? Fourth: how long will it take for the exercise to have a good effect on my health?

The 'Health Through Fitness' schedule on pages 190 – 3 is a guide to an aerobic exercise programme that any able-bodied person can follow and is designed to take the mystery out of aerobic exercise.

If you can, join your local jogging club or aerobics group. If you have any doubts about your health, see your doctor and explain that you are about to take regular exercise. If your doctor thinks that exercise is unhealthy, insist on seeing a doctor who agrees with exercise. The advantage of joining a jogging club or aerobics class is that you should then have access not only to experienced people who can guide you but also to doctors expert in the treatment of fit and healthy people as opposed to ill people. Motivation is the special advantage of a club or group: everybody in the *Fun Runner '82* project agreed that the incentive to keep going was supplied by the teams.

In answer to the first question, there is almost no such thing as an intrinsically aerobic or anaerobic sport or activity. It all depends on how the game is played and on the condition of the player. Because it is too leisurely, cricket is about the only outdoor sport involving activity that is bound to be anaerobic. (For fast bowlers it is anaerobic because the activity is not sustained). Of course, bowls, snooker, darts and similar recreations are not aerobic.

Other sports, such as football, hockey, basketball and squash, are aerobic only if played rather eccentrically, in continuous movement. Men who bring their competitive urges to the squash court and flail around, imagining that sweat and exhaustion are proof against the excesses of their everyday lives, are making a mistake. Squash played that way is anaerobic and will develop speed and strength but not endurance. Also, played fast, it is safe only for the highly fit person; played sporadically by someone with a sedentary job, it is fairly dangerous. Tennis and badminton are, by their nature and if played with some skill, more likely to be aerobic.

By their nature judo, boxing, karate and yoga are unlikely to be aerobic. Circuit training and downhill skiing can only be aerobic for the exceptionally fit person who can keep going without stopping for ten minutes. Weight training can be aerobic only if carried out on special equipment such as Nautilus machines.

If you are a recreational skier you may imagine that you can regularly ski for ten minutes or more without a break. Next time you are on the slopes, time yourself.

The recreations most likely to be aerobic are brisk walking, preferably in hilly country, and dancing. 'Aerobics' is also sometimes called 'aerobic dancing' simply because it is a form of dancing specifically planned to be vigorous for continuous sessions of about ten minutes. Golf can be an aerobic exercise for older people, not when playing a shot but while walking between shots. If a golf cart is used the sport cannot be aerobic. Carry your clubs!

The best aerobic exercise is any exercise that can conveniently be sustained for ten minutes or more at a time. In Britain jogging is the 'best' aerobic exercise simply because it is cheap, convenient and possible any day of the year. (For the beginner, a combination of walking and jogging will be aerobic; for a more experienced person, running.) Swimming is better all-round exercise, because it uses the whole body. The disadvantages of swimming are practical: access to pools, crowds, chlorine, the difficulty of swimming for ten minutes or more without a break. Cross-country ski-ing is the best aerobic exercise of all, and champion cross-country skiers have the highest aerobic capacity of all sportsmen and women.

An out-of-condition sedentary person, perhaps overweight, middle-aged and with a history of breathlessness, may well find any sport or formal exercise too hard at first; brisk walking may be quite taxing. Someone in this condition would certainly be out of breath walking up flights of stairs. If this describes you, be patient! Go for walks of ten minutes and more at your own pace, and don't think of taking vigorous exercise until you feel ready. As the members of *Fun Runner '82*

172

discovered, the body is remarkably resilient and develops quite quickly in response to exercise.

The second question I am most often asked is: 'How can I discover when my heart rate is elevated to sixty to eighty per cent of maximum?' Dr Cooper's estimate of 150 beats a minute applies to younger people, because maximum heart rate is a function of age. Roughly speaking, maximum rate is 220 beats a minute minus your age. For example, at the time of writing I am forty-three years old, so my maximum rate is 177 beats a minute: that is about as fast as my heart will go. Thus younger people have faster maximum rates than older people.

The way to find out whether you are exercising aerobically is to take your pulse, at the wrist or if you prefer at the neck, with a watch with a second hand, immediately after exercise.

This drill is a feature of every well-organised aerobics class. Remember that the exercise should take five minutes at the very minimum: increase it to ten minutes or more as soon as you can. It is best to take your pulse for ten seconds the moment you stop exercising and then multiply by six. Heart rates for people of different ages are as follows:

Age	maximum rate (minute)	60 to 80% rate (minute)	60 to 80% rate (10 seconds)
under 25	200	120 – 160	20 – 27
25 – 29	195	117 – 156	20 – 26
30 – 34	190	114 – 152	19 – 25
35 – 39	185	111 – 148	19 – 25
40 – 44	180	108 – 144	18 – 24
45 – 49	175	105 – 140	18 – 23
50 – 54	170	102 – 136	17 – 23
55 – 59	165	99 – 132	17 – 22
60 – 64	160	96 – 128	16 – 21
65 and over	155	93 – 124	16 – 21

There are two other ways of determining whether exercise is aerobic. Since neither involve a watch or taking the pulse, however, they are less precise. The 'perceived effort' test (also called the 'Borg scale' because it was developed by Gunnar Borg at the University of

Stockholm) requires practice and some self-knowledge. The effort required of exercise is rated on the following scale, from 6 to 20:

6	
7	very, very light
8	
9	very light
10	
11	fairly light
12	
13	somewhat hard
14	
15	hard
16	
17	very hard
18	
19	very, very hard
20	

Aerobic exercise should feel 'somewhat hard' or 'hard', corresponding to 12 – 16 on the scale. This subjective judgement can be verified by checking to see that it relates to a heart rate of 120 – 160 beats a minute. With practice, it is easy to judge without a watch that light or very hard exercise is not aerobic.

The third way of checking whether exercise is aerobic is the 'talk test', which is most useful during a jog. During aerobic exercise you should be able to carry out a conversation, which may be somewhat staccato, with a companion. If you cannot talk during exercise then it cannot be aerobic and will be ineffective; your heart rate is likely to have soared well above 150 beats a minute and you will be in 'oxygen debt'. The result will be that you will have to slow down to an aerobic level of exercise, or stop.

Unfit people often worry unnecessarily about the possible dangers of exercise. The body has ways of foiling people who try too hard. Exhaustion is its first defence. Anybody who persists in exercising too hard is then likely to get injured or depressed. 'Jogger's Blues' is a well-known condition that results from following a training programme designed for an athlete, not an ordinary citizen. Injuries should always be seen as a helpful warning sign. Do not continue to exercise if the pain of an injury gets worse or if the pain is sharp. In such cases see a sympathetic doctor.

To some extent aerobic exercise can be built into a healthy life. Walk to work or to the station; walk up stairs; cycle to work. Some of the women who graduated from the *London 1982/50* and later projects now run to work and have insisted on the installation of showers.

How much exercise?

The third and fourth questions I am most often asked are: 'How long should I exercise, each day and each week?' And: 'How long will it take for the exercise to have a good effect on my health?'

Strictly speaking, the answer to the fourth question is: it depends. The exercise programmes for which I have been responsible – *London 1982/50*, *Fun Runner '82* and, later, the *Sunday Times Getting in Shape* and the *Sisters* projects – have lasted between five months and a year. The most remarkable changes in the completed projects happened about three months after the training began. Men and women of different ages found that their shapes changed (as measured by estimates of body fat, a better gauge than body weight); that they slept better and often needed less sleep; that they enjoyed eating and drinking what they liked; that they gained a natural sense of well-being (and were less inclined to continue with a course of drugs or psychoanalysis); and that they were recovering an enjoyment of their bodies and of playing and striving with other people that they assumed they had lost at the end of childhood.

I asked some participants to tell me what had happened. Michael Innes, a relatively fit twenty-eight-year-old:

Running represents a personal challenge. Eight weeks on from the first tentative steps there has been no great metamorphosis; just a feeling of well-being and a remedy, perhaps, for mental fatigue after a day's work.

Terry Bennett, a forty-one-year-old solicitor who lost a couple of stone observed:

> I love those magic mornings when a mile into the run you feel good, and you know this is a day when you can push yourself almost to your limit for mile after mile, and you finish physically tired but mentally exhilarated.

He was writing about runs in winter, before breakfast and a day's work. Peter Bird, a fifty-seven-year-old insurance underwriter and a veteran of several marathons, had been a diabetic who some years before had decided to save his own life by running. He wrote, of a time when he was four stone heavier:

> I used to roll off the train at Charing Cross in the morning feeling dizzy with high blood pressure. I honestly believe that if I hadn't been encouraged to run, seven years ago, I would be dead by now.

Liz Parry, a twenty-nine-year-old teacher training, not for a marathon, but for the *Fun Run*, wrote:

> I am frankly amazed that I am improving in ways that I thought were personally impossible.

Vivienne Coady, married to a club athlete, enjoyed winning at her own level:

> Once we have put in a couple of miles, I feel really great. I never feel tired; rather, a feeling of being refreshed. When I have felt tired before the run, I no longer feel so, afterwards.

She became a trainer for the *Sunday Times Getting in Shape* project as a way of giving to others what she had got herself. Don Clark, a forty-one-year-old probation officer, ran for another reason, to raise £10,000 for another machine like the one that had saved his life: a long operation had disentangled a cyst from his spinal column. He ran not to save his own life, but those of others. He found that:

> Running is peaceful, and it represents a kind of freedom. It

establishes warm bonds between people. Part of me fell in love with the hippy ideal in the 1960s. The best parts of running allow me to relive the best parts of that.

The reply I enjoyed most came from James Kelly, a forty-nine-year-old local government officer from Swansea:

> I felt lethargic and content to let life pass me by. Then in 1978 I joined in the first Sunday Times National Fun Run. Suddenly I was no longer one of life's spectators. Even the youngest typist was no longer looking at me as if I were her father. Success at last!

People who diet want to stop. People who persevere with an exercise programme do not want to stop.

The answer to the third question is that the Royal College of Physicians recommend twenty minutes of exercise, three times a week. Dr Cooper and Professor Wood have found that lasting health benefits occur at a rather higher level: they both recommend 80 to 120 minutes of exercise a week, preferably in four sessions. For a jogger this is the equivalent of a total of a gentle eight to twelve miles a week, covered perhaps on two days during the week and the two weekend days, the sessions being as evenly spaced as possible. At this level profound changes in the cardiorespiratory system start and continue.

The US Health and Social Services Secretary Richard Schweiker, who had served as a member of the McGovern committee in 1977, said in 1981:

> By taking five simple steps, by not smoking, by using alcohol in moderation, by eating a proper diet and getting the proper amount of exercise and sleep, a forty-five-year-old man can expect to live ten or eleven years longer than a person who does not make these choices.

The hundreds of people of all ages I have run with, talked to, and corresponded with in the last five years have taught me that the first step of these five is exercise. The others follow as a result of exercise. And 'proper diet' turns out to have nothing whatever to do with dieting: for most people who exercise regularly, a proper diet is

177

eating as much good food as they want to eat.

More oxygen; more food

Why is aerobic exercise so special? First of all, because it
is aerobic exercise that speeds up the body and increases
our metabolic rate. Doctors and scientists who have not
found that exercise produces this effect, have not studied
aerobic exercise.

Oxygen is the fuel for our internal fire that burns food.
The more oxygen that is supplied to a flame, the brighter
and faster the flame burns; this is as much true within the
human body as it is within a grate. The action of a bellows
enflames a fire; the action of the lungs, themselves a form
of bellows, sends oxygen into the bloodstream for use in
the conversion of food into energy.

The greater a person's capacity for oxygen, the higher
the metabolic rate of that person will be. The more
oxygen that is supplied, the more food the body can burn.
To be more precise, there is a relationship between the
oxygen intake of a person and the volume of food he or
she requires, in order to be in energy balance. The more
fuel, the bigger the fire.

Food and oxygen combine to make the human fire.
Most studies of energy balance look at food, or at oxygen,
but not both. This makes only limited sense; the body
cannot use one to sustain life without the other. The
reason that the metabolic rate of the person on a diet or a
fast goes down is not a mystery. The body balances a
reduced food intake by reducing oxygen intake, and
reduces oxygen intake still more when energy has to be
taken not from food but from the body itself. Dieters train
their bodies to require less oxygen. The main effect of diet
regimes is to condition the body to tolerate diet regimes,
which it does by a process of adaptation, lowering its
metabolic rate, which is to say its use of oxygen. The
more frequent and more stringent the diet regimes, the
more dramatic and less reversible these effects will be.

It also follows that the body will balance a greater
intake of food by taking in more oxygen, up to the point
at which it has no more capacity. A very big man who is

also phenomenally physically active will therefore have a gigantic appetite, but when as a result of change of habits or age or infirmity he ceases to exercise, much of the food he eats will turn to fat. This is because less exercise means less oxygen taken in, and less oxygen taken in means that energy balance can be sustained only if less food is eaten. Hence the dramatic fattening of Henry VIII and Edward VII when they stopped hunting.

The analogy with a fire in a grate is fair. Suitably ventilated, a small amount of coal burns bright and low; a large amount of coal burns bright and high. If a bellows is applied to a small amount of coal, more will soon be needed. If, on the other hand, little air can get to either a small or a large amount of coal, it will burn low, or not be burned at all.

Scientific studies of under-nutrition and over-nutrition are the key to understanding what dieting does to the human body. The body's use of the fuel, oxygen, varies as a function of the body's use of the fuel, food. As well as food, the body itself contains another fuel: fat. Just as food is burned with oxygen, fat is burned with oxygen. Dieting lowers the body's capacity for oxygen. Dieting therefore lowers the body's capacity to burn its own fat; it is stored, instead.

The study of energy balance is the study not only of balance between energy taken in as food and energy used, but also of the balance between energy taken in from food and energy taken in from oxygen. In the energy equation, oxygen is not a 'given', a constant; it is a variable.

When energy from food outbalances energy from oxygen, fat is stored, and obesity is the result. Dieting reduces energy from oxygen, and so is self-defeating. Over-eating increases energy from oxygen, which is, however, outbalanced by the extra energy taken in from food. The way out of this circle is to take in more energy without taking in more food: to apply the bellows of the lungs to the body's fire.

The muscle that uses fat as fuel

Sustained aerobic exercise results in loss of fat and gain of lean tissue. In time its 'training effect' increases the metabolic activity of the muscles at all times. Another reason why aerobic rather than anaerobic exercise has this effect is that the two types of exercise use different types of muscle. There are two types of muscle fibre: red muscle fibre (also known as 'slow-twitch' muscle), used for work requiring endurance; and white muscle fibre (also known as 'fast-twitch' muscle), used for work requiring immediate reaction. Aerobic exercise uses red muscle, anaerobic exercise white muscle.

It is not known to what extent, if at all, exercise can alter the proportions of red and white muscle. It is known that some people are 'red muscle types', meaning that their muscles contain a relatively high proportion of red fibres; and other people are 'white muscle types', meaning that their muscles contain a relatively high proportion of white fibres. To take runners as an example: sprinters are white muscle types, constantly using fast-twitch fibre for explosive action; marathoners are red muscle types, constantly using slow-twitch fibre for their methodical long-distance running.

The fuel used by white muscle fibre is glycogen; naturally enough, because glycogen is the body's immediately available source of energy, and can be instantly mobilised by muscle in action. The glycogen store is essential and is replaced after the white muscle fibres have done their anaerobic work, together with the water bound up with it. Anaerobic activity does not burn fat. This is why it is physically impossible to lose fat, or indeed to lose weight except temporarily, if your style of playing squash is to thrash around the court anaerobically.

Red muscle fibre also uses glycogen as fuel. But, to take the analogy of a domestic fire, it does so not as its main fuel, but as kindling. The equivalent of coal – slow-burning, releasing much energy – for red muscle, is body fat. To be more precise, red muscle fibre uses fat released from the body's stores into the bloodstream, in the form of a liquid, free fatty acid. The fat store of the body is of course there, to be used as fuel, and unlike glycogen does not need to be replaced.

It is aerobic exercise – endurance work – that uses red muscle, and hence fat, as fuel. This is common sense.

180

Aerobic exercise corresponds to the necessary work done by people who do not live in industrialised societies, such as Eskimos and Bushmen; or remote peoples such as Lapps; or peasants in the West, such as the country people of the Swiss Alps. These people do not gain weight or fat throughout their lives; they work aerobically at regular intervals; and they eat well. Even the most athletic hunter does not very often do the equivalent of playing squash. It is constant walking that wears away a stone or two.

Just like any machine that is neglected and rusted, the function of the human body degenerates with disuse. Sedentary adults who fondly imagine that it is only dignity that prevents them gambolling about, as they did when children, should have a try when no one is looking: they will have an unpleasant surprise.

A machine that is carefully tended and oiled will preserve its usefulness. Here, though, the human body is unlike a machine: for the body actually improves with use. This is conspicuously the case with muscle.

Muscles need oxygen. Aerobic training develops the flow of oxygen within muscle, and this in turn develops the functioning of the muscle. In particular, the 'training effect' created by three to six months' aerobic exercise (for most able-bodied people) develops the ability of muscle to use fat as fuel. In their classic *Textbook of Work Physiology* Per-Olof Åstrand and Kaare Rodahl put it as follows:

> Since the ability to utilise fat as a fuel depends on the oxygen transporting capacity, the choice of fuel for the working muscle depends on the workload in relation to the individual's maximal oxygen uptake. The greater the maximal oxygen uptake, the greater the percentage contribution of fat to the energy metabolism at a given workload. Since training increases the maximal oxygen uptake, it also increases the facility for utilising fat as a source of muscular energy.

Professor Åstrand has written to me to confirm that sustained aerobic training not only develops the ability of red muscle to use fat as fuel, but also develops some such potential in white muscle. The human body is marvellously responsive to the positively beneficial stress put upon it by regular, vigorous exercise. And so, the way

181

to develop the body's capacity to use fat as fuel, is constantly to exercise in a way that requires fat as fuel: aerobically.

Conversely, it is idle to suppose that muscle will remain in good shape if, after childhood, the body becomes inactive. Our bodies are in a state of constant modification, throughout life. The muscle fibre of sedentary people becomes increasingly shot through with fat, just like the marbled steak from a steer kept artificially penned up, so as to provide juicy, fatty meat.

Is there hope for very fat people?

The muscle fibre of sedentary people, who use less and less oxygen, adjusts so as to use less and less oxygen. With this, sedentary people gradually lose the wherewithal to burn fat. Some new evidence suggests that, with long disuse, red muscle degenerates into a white-type muscle, so losing the function of using body fat as fuel. If this is so, it explains why doctors who work with very obese patients state that exercise is ineffective as a means of weight control. It also explains why the three very overweight women who completed the *Fun Runner '82* project got fitter but, paradoxically, did not lose weight and lost little fat.

Experienced and conscientious doctors who work with grossly obese patients, more often than not form the view – privately, if not publicly – that obesity is intractable. Jaw-wiring, or semi-starvation regimes over a period of perhaps a year in hospital conditions, achieve massive weight loss. But, as with 'Weight Watcher Of The Year' or 'Slimmer Of The Year' contests, most very obese people who lose remarkable amounts of weight, regain their fat, and more, in time.

It is possible that some very obese people have indeed irreversibly lost the means to use fat as fuel. There comes a point with various diseases and disorders, when damage cannot be made good. Faced with the choice of surgery or philosophy, the wise choice is, like Falstaff, to make the best of a big and burgeoning body.

But it is probable that the majority of people who are

over-fat, even very over-fat, can reverse their state by means of exercise. First, it is a question of understanding that the process by which the naturally active body of childhood is liable to become fat when adult and sedentary, is a slow, long process, not reversible by a week or three months' regime. Moreover, the process whereby relatively inactive fat is replaced by active lean tissue will discourage those who rely on their bathroom scales, simply because muscle is heavier than fat. The measurement to take, as you start to exercise and so regenerate your body, is of your waist, not your weight. And be patient!

If your purpose in exercising is not only to become fit, but also to lose fat, there is increasing evidence that the secret is not intensity, but duration, of exercise. Dr Eric Newsholme of Oxford University, a biochemist who is currently working on new research on this subject, is inclined to believe that the body contains what might be termed a 'fat-burning mechanism' which is switched on only after maybe half-an-hour of exercise.

If Dr Newsholme is right, and my own experience and that of the people I have worked with suggests that he is, then the motto for people who want to lose fat is: keep going. My recommendation for sedentary out of shape adults, especially if over thirty-five, is: long walks, first of all. These walks will be aerobic, if they are vigorous enough to work up a sweat; and they will be good for the waistline, after three months or so – sometimes sooner – if they last half an hour or more, with no stops.

The new enthusiasm for jogging and running, which I share, may have the unfortunate effect, for some people, of discouraging them from taking less vigorous – and less conspicuous – forms of exercise. Few women over the age of thirty-five look forward to the prospect of running in singlet and shorts. Citizens do not get medals for walking – even for the marathon distance of twenty-six and more miles – but if your purpose, in taking exercise, is to lose fat, it may very well be that the positively most effective method is to walk long distances rather than run for a couple of miles. And walking, especially in the countryside at weekends, can be a way to enjoy fresh air and the company of your family, or at least your dog.

I foresee a time when positive health centres are established throughout Britain, with the purpose of encouraging citizens to realise their full potential, by means of health tests followed by individual advice on food and exercise. Meanwhile, long vigorous walks will not only trim your waistline, but also enliven the functions of your gut and encourage a sense of natural well-being.

What about hunger? Many people are put off exercise because they find that, afterwards, they feel ravenously hungry. Writers who favour exercise tend to claim that, for reasons which are unclear to them, exercise does not make you hungry. My experience is that most people who take exercise scoff at such claims; usually, exercise makes you hungry, all right. So how can exercise have the effect of losing weight?

As you start to exercise, regularly and vigorously, remember that aerobic exercise speeds up your metabolic rate throughout the day. After a while you will notice the difference: people who have progressed from being basically sedentary to being active, wear fewer clothes, take blankets off the bed and sleep with a window open, stop suffering from cold hands and feet, and generally feel warmer all the time. That's what having a higher metabolic rate means, in terms of everyday experience. So don't worry about feeling hungry. Eat! The secret, though, is to eat whole, bulky foods, full of nourishment, and to lay off foods saturated with processed sugar and fat. There are few meals more satisfying than a steaming hot vegetable stew, with meat too if you like, on the day of a long walk or run. My own favourite is ratatouille. Offal like oxtail is delicious in a stew, too.

Remember, too, that aerobic exercise loses fat and gains lean tissue. Do not expect to lose weight; you may, or may not, in the first three or so months. Instead, measure your waistline (and other parts of your body, as shown on page 193). Enjoy a little ceremony: burn all the calorie charts you have in the house, and then put your bathroom scales in the dustbin.

Dr Newsholme's investigations may, however, explain why some physiologists have found that exercise does not make you hungry. The fitter you are, and the more exercise you take, the more your body is trained, during aerobic exercise, to burn its own fat. But this fat burning mechanism, Dr Newsholme proposes, switches on after half-an-hour or so of exercise. It follows that any exercise taking less than half-an-hour, whether or not it is aerobic, will only use glycogen as fuel. And since hunger is signalled when glycogen stores are low, it also follows that an exercise of any type lasting under half-an-hour or so will have the effect of making you hungry; whereas relatively gentle exercise, at the bottom end of the aerobic range, will have the effect of supplying energy from body fat and so make you less hungry.

This hypothesis certainly corresponds with my own experience. For me, a short run of four miles makes me hungry; whereas after a long weekend run of maybe fifteen miles, or two hours or more, I do not feel like a meal. Moreover, I have often noticed a 'third wind' after thirty to forty minutes into a run, which might be the fat-burning mechanism 'switching on'. Dr. Newsholme's proposals are backed by his own experience of progressing from a sedentary sixteen and a half stone to a twelve and a half stone marathon runner. It will take a number of years for some of the most exciting scientific work being done in the fields of food and exercise to be proved. Meanwhile, good advice to anyone who has decided to become fit and healthy is: trust your own experience.

Aerobic exercise is the most effective treatment for the most common disorders of the gut. I have never come across a constipated jogger. It's my opinion, too, that aerobic exercise is the most effective first step to positive health, because, as with the 'Fun Runner '82' members, regular exercise brings with it an appetite for good whole food. I have lost count of the number of people, who now take regular exercise, who have said to me: I really used to look forward to cream buns and doughnuts and chocolate eclairs – but now, I think I fancy them, but I don't. My own version of this experience, was the first time I ran eighteen miles: four circuits of Hyde Park and Kensington Gardens. The last lap was very painful, and I kept going by having thoughts of the fudge ice-cream and coffee eclairs I'd buy on Queensway, and then devour, as my reward. In the event, I threw these treats away: I couldn't stomach them. They were too sweet, too 'rich'.

If aerobic exercise damps down the desire for processed sugar, then it is a vital preventive of, and treatment for, diabetes. That is the view of Professor Michael Berger, a leading specialist in diabetes. Any diabetic whose pancreas is destroyed will of course have to go on injecting insulin. But almost all diabetics, including children, have a pancreas which is damaged but not destroyed; and Dr Berger has found that his patients respond to regular exercise. Indeed, he has found that diabetic children, who are often told that exercise is dangerous, are at risk not from exercise, but from the insulin they inject, which becomes an overdose when combined with exercise. The answer, is to exercise and take a much lower dose of insulin.

The way, therefore, to prevent a pre-diabetic state, is to exercise and eat good food. And the way to allow a pre-diabetic state, or a condition diagnosed as adult-onset diabetes, to recede, is, likewise, to exercise and eat good food. Western doctors are not noted for explaining the cause and cure of Western diseases. Western diseases are caused by inactivity and bad food, principally. There comes a point, with any severe disease, when it is irreversible; before that point, however, it can be reversed, or at least quietened, simply by using the body well. In the case of diabetes, obviously the best means to mend and nourish the pancreas, is to behave in a way which will allow it to restore its natural function; which is to say, by eating the best food for non-diabetic people: whole food rich in starch, protein fibre, vitamins and minerals, and no processed sugar.

The revolution in modern medicine is being created by doctors, scientists, therapists and experienced people who have come to realise that, in the long view, the way to prevent and to treat Western diseases, is exactly the same as the way to encourage positive health for people who are not ill: by means of plenty of fresh air and plenty of good food. It is only our fascination with technology that prevents us realising what doctors down the ages always knew.

The effects of aerobic exercise on the function of the heart, lungs and blood vessels are well known. With sustained aerobic exercise, say for sessions totalling 80 to 120 minutes a week, the blood vessels enlarge and become more elastic. The heart, itself a muscle, becomes stronger and larger. Blood pressure drops. A further consequence is that resting heart rate drops, from say, the 'average' seventy-two beats a minutes, to sixty and then down even further, to maybe fifty.

Trained athletes often have a heart rate in the forties. The average heart rate of the *London 1982/50* participants dropped to the fifties after marathon training. The simplest test of a healthy heart is resting heart rate; and it is very satisfying, knowing this, to find that heart rate drops, steadily, during a course of aerobic training.

At the same time, the heart also pumps more blood. Dr Kenneth Cooper estimates that aerobically trained people will have up to two extra pints of blood in their bodies. This is because of a process of 'vascularisation' whereby blood vessels not only enlarge but also grow in number. The blood vessels on the surface of the heart itself become larger and more elastic, and are therefore far less likely to be the site of a heart attack. Thomas Bassler, an American doctor, once claimed that running marathons gave anyone without a pre-existing heart condition 100 per cent protection against a fatal heart attack caused by irreversible blockage within a blood vessel. This claim is disputed, but there is no doubt that a runner's cardiovascular system is stronger than that of a non-runner.

It is healthier as well as stronger. Professor Wood, supported by other studies, has shown that high proportions of the abrasive, useful HDL lipoprotein are associated with aerobic exercise equivalent to jogging eight to twelve miles a week. Below that level, exercise does not have a great effect on blood lipid levels. In California anyone can buy a customised car registration number: Professor Wood's is HIGH HDL, to remind people in the car behind of the good effects of running. Cholesterol is not in itself a health hazard. It is the type of fat in the blood that determines whether or not someone is at risk, and sedentary people tend to have high levels of the sticky LDL lipoprotein in their blood.

Aerobic exercise also promotes the growth of blood vessels close to the surface of the skin. This accounts for the healthy glow of runners and encourages rejuvenation of the skin. There is also evidence that aerobic exercise slows down or even reverses the tendency of bone to become decalcified and so brittle with age. Old people who break their bones as a result of a fall are usually sedentary people. According to the Royal College of Physicians:

> The need for middle-aged and elderly people to continue to engage in regular and substantial periods of moderate activity each week runs counter to current practice . . . There seems little doubt that the majority of adults in sedentary occupations are physiologically 'unfit' with poor cardiovascular responses to exercises.

Reasons for the exercise 'high'

New research is being done on the relationship of aerobic exercise and endorphin levels. Only recently identified and traced, endorphins are chemical substances whose structure is similar to morphine. Consequently they are sometimes known as 'the body's natural opiates'. There is some evidence that endorphin pathways are the pathways traced by acupuncturists, and so account for the otherwise mysterious anaesthetic effect of acupuncture.

Endorphins are released by the body under exercise – or induced stress – and may postpone the sensation of pain in physical crisis until the need for action has passed. They may be what enables a footballer with a broken collar-bone to score a goal, or a runner to complete a race with blisters.

There is evidence that smoking inhibits the flow of endorphins, replacing this natural process with the artificial soothing of nicotine; hence smoking's addictive qualities. There is also evidence that aerobic exercise 'jogs' the endorphins into action. So the way of stopping smoking may be to start aerobic exercise, not try to give up smoking, and see what happens. Half the *London 1982/50* and *Fun Runner '82* participants who started as smokers found that they stopped more or less spontaneously during the projects. They found themselves instead enjoying the 'jogger's high', the natural and intense sense of well-being of which endorphins are the source. Hence Terry Bennett's 'magic mornings'.

For people who are out of shape aerobic exercise is the way forward. Dieting will only depress an overweight person. We need more air. Aerobic exercise allows us to eat more while losing fat. In moderation, it puts the body in energy balance at a natural level, higher than that of a sedentary person, so that good food can provide enough nourishment. Aerobic exercise enlivens the alimentary tract and strengthens the cardiovascular system. It is the means to health through fitness.

Table 4. Health Through Fitness

This aerobic training schedule is based on ten rules, seven stages, and forty-nine steps to be taken at your own pace, as it suits you. It will work for all able-bodied people whatever their initial state of fitness. Remember that it takes a long time for the body to get out of shape; so it will take some months to regain what you have lost.

The Ten Rules

1. *Start at the beginning.* Whatever your initial state of fitness start at stage 1. Do not move up a stage until you can complete every session in a week comfortably.

2. *Variety is the spice.* Some sessions are longer, moving from 10 to 40 minutes from stages 1 – 7; others are shorter, building up from 5 – 10 to 20 – 30 minutes.

3. *Rest as well as exercise.* Start with three and then four sessions a week, as shown, with rest days in between. (The chart assumes that weekend days are convenient; if not, of course other days will do as well.)

4. *One step and stage at a time.* Progress at your own pace. Don't force yourself to move from one stage to the next. The best test of your progress is a sense of well-being and energy after exercise.

5. *Backsliding is OK.* If you find a stage too hard, move back. If you get fed up or ill for a while, don't worry. Start a stage below where you left off. You will enjoy holidays more if you keep exercising.

6. *Train aerobically.* Walk-jogging, then jogging, is the most reliable aerobic exercise: it is simple, available, easy to measure. The two longer sessions should be jogging. For the other sessions please yourself with any aerobic exercise.

7 *Measure your own fitness.* At the very beginning, and every time you move up a stage, measure your fitness (by means of the system on page 193).

8. *First target is 80 – 120 minutes a week.* Stages 5 – 7 are where the cardiovascular benefits will take place, provided that your exercise is aerobic.

9. *Second target is 8 – 12 miles a week*. As soon as you reach stage 5, you are ready for the 'two-mile' test on p. 193. Use this to check that you are, when you jog, covering 8 – 12 miles a week or its equivalent in other aerobic exercise.

10. *Warm up and warm down*. Before and after every session stretch and bend your body, and jog on the spot or walk, for a few minutes.

There is no rule about how long it will take to reach stage 5: it all depends on you. If you treat the schedule as a competition and push yourself up stages you are fairly likely to injure yourself. As a rough guide, the majority of people I have worked with have taken ten to twenty weeks to reach stage 5. If you reach stage 7 and want to go further, see 'Further Reading' on page 249.

The Seven Stages and The 49 Steps

	Sat	Sun	Mon	Tues	Wed	Thurs	Fri	Total
Stage 1	10	—	—	5	—	5	—	20
Stage 2	15	—	—	5	—	10	—	30
Stage 3	20	—	—	10	—	10	—	40
Stage 4	25	10	—	10	—	15	—	60
Stage 5	30	15	—	15	—	20	—	80
Stage 6	35	15	—	25	—	25	—	100
Stage 7	40	20	—	30	—	30	—	120

Days printed in bold are the days for jogging. All days left blank are rest days. The rest days are a vital part of the forty-nine steps. The figures are minutes. As long as the total for the week is right you can vary the length of any session, but do not shorten the long run and do not cut out sessions.

What this schedule is designed to do, is to give you a framework for your own schedule, which you can design to suit yourself. Just make sure that your own schedule follows the ten rules, above.

You may well want to base your own schedule on aerobics classes (or dance/exercise, popmobility, etc). If these classes are really and truly aerobic (pages 170 – 175) then include them as part of your schedule. But often 'aerobics' classes are not really aerobic: test them. In any case, don't rely completely on classes. In the long term the most effective aerobic exercise is vigorous walking, graduating to jogging and running, simply because exercise is readily sustained at a steady 60 – 80 per cent of maximum heart rate.

The sense of physical and mental well-being that grows, with aerobic exercise, is as good an indication of the development of health through fitness as any test a doctor can perform.

You will find it valuable and fascinating to measure the development of your health through fitness, by the tests opposite. Carry them out every time you reach a new stage in the Seven-Stage plan.

The 'self-measurement' tests on the chart, you can carry out yourself. The way to measure your heart rate at rest and after exercise is explained on pp. 173-4. The 'fitness tests' are offered at some health clubs and doctors' clinics. Search them out.

When you reach stage 5 find out how long it takes you to run two miles. Eight laps of an athletic track is near enough two miles; otherwise prepare a route on a large-scale map. Do the 'two-mile' test every month once you reach stage 5.

Gear. You will need shoes especially made for jogging. These have built-up heels and look a bit like landing craft. They are expensive. Do not skimp on them; they prevent injuries to the lower legs and knees. You will also need a tracksuit for cold days, and of course shorts and T-shirts.

Diary. You will find it very helpful to keep a diary in which you enter every exercise session, together with notes on the weather, your state of health at the time, how you felt, length of exercise session, and so on. As time goes on and you get fitter a diary is great for motivation, and as a means to pay attention to your body. You might like to make copies of the 'self measurement' tests and insert them in your diary.

Clubs and classes. Jogging clubs are springing up all over the country, and some established running clubs now welcome beginners. Likewise, aerobics classes are growing at a great rate. Clubs or classes are also great for motivation, and can be good fun too. Find them in your locality by contacting your local health education officer, sports/leisure centre, or even, in some enlightened cities like Oxford, the town hall.

Magazines. The new specialist magazines, most of which are new, regularly carry details of clubs, classes, new ideas, fitness testing centres, and so forth. For the jogger and runner the magazine is 'Fitness'. For everybody with an interest in fitness, health and good food, the magazine is 'New Health.' If you want to contact me, write to 'New Health' at 38 – 42 Hampton Road, Teddington, Middlesex TW11 0JE, enclosing a stamped addressed envelope.

Self-measurement

	Start	Stages:						
		1	2	3	4	5	6	7
Body (inches)								
Chest/Bust	__	__	__	__	__	__	__	__
Waist	__	__	__	__	__	__	__	__
Hips	__	__	__	__	__	__	__	__
Thighs	__	__	__	__	__	__	__	__
Weight (pounds)	__	__	__	__	__	__	__	__
Heart Rate (per minute)								
At rest	__	__	__	__	__	__	__	__
After exercise[1]	__	__	__	__	__	__	__	__
3 minutes after	__	__	__	__	__	__	__	__
10 minutes after	__	__	__	__	__	__	__	__
Two Mile Test								
Minutes/seconds taken	__	__	__	__	__	__	__	__
Fitness Tests								
Blood Pressure	__	__	__	__	__	__	__	__
Body Fat Percentage	__	__	__	__	__	__	__	__
Oxygen Capacity[2]	__	__	__	__	__	__	__	__
Fitness Rating[3]	__	__	__	__	__	__	__	__

[1] immediately afterwards
[2] VO_2 Max (ml O_2 min kg)
[3] Cooper scales

The charts and schedule on these pages were designed in consultation with Will Chapman, Dr Kenneth Cooper, Malcolm Emery, Tom McNab and Professor Peter Wood.

CHAPTER SIX

The Woman Dieter

> In this era, when inflation has assumed alarming
> proportions and the threat of nuclear war has become a
> serious danger, when violent crime is on the increase and
> unemployment a persistent social fact, 500 people are
> asked by the pollsters what they fear most in the world and
> 190 answer that their greatest fear is 'getting fat'.
> KIM CHERNIN
> *The Obsession*

> 'I suppose you really do believe that your happiness is
> consequent on your size? That an inch or two one way or
> the other would make you truly loved? Equating prettiness
> with sexuality, and sexuality with happiness? It is a very
> debased view of sexuality you take, Phyllis. It would be
> excusable in a 16-year-old – if my nose were a different
> shape, if my bosom were larger, if my freckles were gone,
> then the whole world would be different. But in a woman
> of your age it is vulgar.'
> FAY WELDON
> *The Fat Woman's Joke*

Fat is seen as wrong

Fear of becoming fat and desire to lose weight obsess
women in the West. As the Duchess of Windsor said, 'A
woman can never be too rich, or too thin.' In our society
being slim is associated with glamour, success and beauty.
Slimness is felt to be the ideal to which all women should
aspire. The image of the fat man retains an attraction, as an
embodiment of power (Winston Churchill) or of joviality
(Falstaff). But the image of the fat woman, the 'earth

mother', has been rejected, in a culture that has turned away from the virtues she represents.

It is harder for women to deviate from society's ideals. Fat women are penalised far more than fat men. Fat girls are less likely to gain college places than thin girls, they are less likely to be given help of any kind, they are more likely – even than the disabled – to be rejected socially. And they cannot find fashionable clothes that fit them.

Fat is seen as wrong at a very early age. In 1978 three researchers from the University of Cincinnati College of Medicine presented a group of pre-school children with two life-size rag dolls, identical except in one respect – and found that ninety-one per cent of the children preferred the thin doll to the fat doll. And they also found that, although the small number of overweight children in the group correctly identified themselves as looking like the fat doll, they all preferred the thin doll.

In the same study the children were presented with line drawings of children of their own age, varying according to weight, sex and age: for example, a fat white girl, a fat black girl, a thin white boy. The children were asked to pick out which drawings they 'especially liked' or 'disliked' and those they thought were 'weak', 'happy', and so on.

All the children preferred the thin children. The investigators wrote: 'There were three substantial trends: to see fat girls and thin boys as anti-social, to rate boys as more competent than girls, and to describe thin children as more competent than fat children.' In other words, their peers mark out fat girls as inept and unattractive long before they have a chance to prove their talents and sociability at school and later.

After a study undertaken in 1963 the nutritionist Professor Jean Mayer stated:

> When obese subjects demonstrate attitudes similar to those resulting from ethnic and racial prejudice, it is not far-fetched to say that obese persons may form a minority group suffering from prejudice and discrimination.

Women's fear of becoming fat, and their perennial dieting, spring from sources deeper than taste or fashion. In our society only thin is good.

A personal tale

I became a devotee of the cult of slenderness when I was nineteen, in my first year at university. I come from a European family whose eating habits are un-English; at school, a London mixed comprehensive, we brought our own sandwiches for lunch, or went out. I expected great things from university. What I got – among other things – was my first experience of institutional cooking and communal eating. It was a shock.

In the first term, we had to eat breakfast in college. I was appalled, fascinated too, by the cornflakes, greasy fried eggs, mounds of baked beans and floppy white bread. I did what was expected of me, and tucked in. And in a strange new world, for those first lonely few weeks, food was comforting. I felt sick and stodgy quite a lot of the time, but I had been brought up to eat up; mealtimes in my family were a recognised source of pleasure.

In eight weeks I gained ten pounds. I was horrified. For the first time in my life I felt gross.

I came to loathe the smell of stewed cabbage and gravy, and began to associate the grey lukewarm meals with the girls who ate them. I shrank from the image I saw of hundreds of pasty faces wolfing down fodder. My fear, I now recognise, was of being swallowed up by the mass, of losing my own identity.

Eating punctuated every occasion. The cakes, the chocolate, the teas and biscuits, the late-night cocoa, the furtive and not-so-furtive Mars Bars and Kit-Kats, as essays were written or confidences swapped! We were lonely and unhappy girls, stuck out in remote and draughty buildings, eating as compensation, not for pleasure. I was disgusted and miserable. One day there was only one pair of trousers I could wear. I panicked. This was not, could not be me. I had – I decided with compulsive urgency – to reject this environment.

I needed an image, an identity, that worked for me and was as distinct from those around me as possible. And so I decided to get thin. Returning for the second term, I began my campaign. I still remember my first evening back. I announced that I 'didn't want' dinner and went to bed early with a mug of hot milk, feeling excited, empty and

196

nervous. I had been brought up to eat properly; this was a whole new experience.

I became good at calorie counting. Soon I knew the energy content of scores of foods by heart. Fruit, yoghurt, crispbread and endless cottage cheese; salads; picnics in friends' rooms: these became my eating routine. As often as not conversation revolved around food and slimming. I read slimming magazines. Proper sit-down meals made me nervous. Life was busy. I cycled everywhere, and I became addicted to the process of slimming. I swung from highs to lows; from feeling on top, beautiful, in control, to troughs of feeling depressed, weak, defeated. I came to associate the lows with 'feeling fat', and forced myself back to ever fiercer self-denial.

After a few days' fasting I would go back to my mouse portions of cheese and crispbread, with 'rewards' of chocolate. When I did go out to dinner, the next day was a day of penance. I loved being skinny. It was the mark of my self-control and my 'headiness'. I wore tight jeans and a navy Guernsey for nearly all my four university years to emphasise my streamlined image. And I was encouraged by other girls' remarks. 'How thin you are!' they said. I heard envy and admiration.

I wasn't aware how thin I had become; I rarely weighed myself. When my jeans were tight, I felt fat; as long as I remained at size ten I was happy. I'm five foot seven and a half; at that time I weighed eight stone eight pounds, sometimes as little as eight stone three. I suppose I approached the state of anorexia nervosa. But I did eat regularly, even if the quantities were tiny, and I did eat meals when avoiding them would have meant embarrassment or confrontation – at home, for instance. Nevertheless over a period of six years I became very attached to my own habits, always preferring a snack to a meal – which also meant eating cake or a biscuit, as well as fruit, rather than something substantial cooked. My unexpressed fear was that if I ate normal meals regularly I would lose control, be swamped by my body.

I realise now that I kept myself permanently under-nourished. Looking back, my high times were memorable. But they were peaks rising from valleys of depression, listlessness, body-weariness. I got cold very easily. My digestion was bad. I suffered from anxiety. I suppose I assumed that these malaises were the human condition, woman's condition, or my personal bad luck. It did not occur to me that dieting was making me ill. I thought that to be thin was to be healthy – by definition, almost.

Later on in London, no longer living alone, I could not avoid meals. Gradually and with some pain, I began to recognise my fear of food as a neurosis. My obsession with a super-slim profile began to fade, but it took a long time to stop panicking as I put on weight, to stop assuming that I would be judged and rejected in terms of my weight, to stop putting an image before the needs, health and fitness of my body.

And I began to see, too, the irony of the obsession that so many women have with their weight today. It is taken for granted that to be attractive women must be slim. How remarkable that, at a time when women have never been freer to express their opinions and exercise their rights, they are most bound to constrain the shape and weight of their bodies, by dieting.

Fear of fatness

The 1983 Royal College of Physicians' report on obesity cites a recent estimate that, at any one time, sixty-five per cent of British women are trying to lose weight; and that of the thirty-one per cent of the population who are regular users of one or more slimming products, most are women.

Statistics indicate the extent of dieting. They cannot convey the emotional involvement or the cost in terms of money, time, energy and pain. The 1982 report of the *Economist Intelligence Unit* on health products states that slimming is no longer to be seen as a special activity separate from normal eating. We have moved, the EIU report claims, 'towards the concept of weight management as part of regular personal health care'. But for women, dieting is less a question of 'weight management' or 'health care', more a way of life.

Clair Chapman is an actress with the Spare Tyre Theatre Company, a British comedy cabaret group whose acts comment on the state of women and their bodies. Interviewed in December 1981 she said: 'I was put on a diet by my mother when I was twelve. Dieting was an initiation into womanhood. I thought women just had periods and dieted.'

Many women have come to know the cycle of dieting and relapse, pounds lost and pounds regained, as intimately as they know their menstrual cycle. The discomfort of self-denial is followed by the guilt of eating again, and the body gradually becomes more and more flabby, not just in the mind, but in reality.

Katina Noble, another actress with Spare Tyre, said:

> I remember how humiliated I was when my boyfriend said I must get some weight off before we went on a holiday abroad. How desperate I felt, on going to a hypnotist and finding a money-grabbing charlatan. After eight years of this I was just so neurotic. I went up and down between 8½ and 12 stone, but I was just as suicidal at 9 stone 4 as I was at 11 stone 12. I went to such lengths to cover up! Making sure the upper arms weren't showing, never showing my bottom, not wearing trousers for six or seven years; I used to wear a skirt down to my ankles. My whole life was piles of clothes.

A turning-point precipitates many women into the dieting cycle. Very often this turning-point is adolescence, fear of the sudden curves, thighs and breasts of womanhood. Sometimes the crisis is pregnancy when the body not only contains another being but also gains weight fast. Postnatal depression compounds the alienation a mother may feel from her own body, and she may throw herself into a diet which fights her needs and those of her baby at just the time when, if she is breast-feeding, she most needs proper and nourishing food.

Other women diet because of approaching middle age. They refuse to accept that youth is past and focus on being slim as a way of showing that they remain attractive. For these women ageing is to be feared, in a society that prefers the freshness of youth to the wisdom of years. So often in middle age women subject themselves to chronic under-nutrition and lose their self-esteem.

Why do we see only slim women as beautiful? Why are anorexia nervosa and other eating disorders increasing?

Why has dieting mania gone so far that the top 'non-fiction' best-sellers are diet books, in the USA and now in Great Britain as well? Why are women so uncomfortable with food and their bodies?

The woman as provider

Traditionally, women have been denied the power to shape and control their lives. But they have enjoyed sovereignty in two areas: food and nurture, and beauty and the body.

Food, feeding, feasting, eating, cultivation, harvest: these are all concepts rich in meaning and ritual. Notwithstanding our mechanised world of fast food chains, baked beans and packet mash, everything that food stands for retains its symbolic meaning much more than we may care to realise. To offer food is still a primary act of hospitality, acceptance and love. And the principal responsibility for feeding, as for all other forms of nurture, has always fallen to women. The first food of life comes naturally from the mother's own body.

It is the woman who shops, cooks, feeds her man and her children. It is her responsibility to make food wholesome and appetising. Every day she provides for her family. Yet our culture teaches her to beware of feeding herself. Next to recipes for mouth-watering meals, magazines print the latest diet instructions. In one feature women are taught to create a miracle of meringue and cream; in the next to avoid the temptation of puddings.

What happens to a woman brought up on this double-think? Many become adepts. Others become what are now termed 'compulsive eaters': they eat neurotically, either too much or too little, in response to signals that have little to do with real hunger or appetite. These women become out of touch with their real needs and desires; their sense of control over the process of feeding themselves becomes shaky and intermittent.

Women who restrict themselves to 1000 to 1500 calories a day subject themselves to voluntary semi-starvation. The diet ended, the woman (and a male dieter too) is liable to fall on food with an intense and insatiable hunger that persists for a remarkably long time. This is why the dieter, ending the prison-like sentence of the regime, so often celebrates with what may very well be the first of another series of binges. But even if the dieter does not over-eat, in due course the old weight is regained.

Thus are the seeds sown for compulsive over-eating: uncontrolled eating of entire gateaux, quarts of ice-cream, shelves-full of food from the refrigerator, by night as well as by day. The dieter is aware of what is happening, finds no way to stop, and is full of despair.

The new religion

These cycles of denial and reward, starvation and gorging, are familiar to many seasoned dieters. In *Fat is a Feminist Issue* Susie Orbach says that American women spend $10 billion a year on weight control methods. There are five chains of slimming clubs in Great Britain, all thriving, and more in the USA. In the United Kingdom, Weightwatchers alone runs 1400 classes every week. In the USA the Diet Workshop runs 14,000 groups where 45,000 people meet weekly. Late in 1982 *People* magazine reported on the Cambridge Diet, a soluble powder sold at mass rallies by 177,000 'counsellors' throughout the USA who make $6 on every $20 can.

> One after another they rose to testify. 'We are part of a fresh spring rain to wash clean the body of mankind' enthused one of the faithful. 'He is Julius Caesar' wept a follower, referring to the leader. 'He is everything! Isn't he gorgeous! Our leaders do love us! This is a magnificent church!'

Dieting is taking on the forms of religion: churches, prophets, bishops, priests, confession, surrender, redemption, and communion celebrated not with bread and wine, the symbols of an age-old meal, but with chemicals. Slimming clubs report that ninety per cent of their clientele are women. The readership of slimming magazines is similar. *Slimming*, once published and edited by Audrey Eyton, author of *The F-Plan Diet*, and the most successful of the six British slimming magazines, has a circulation of 321,000.

Women's therapy centrês have now been founded in London and New York. The Centre in London reports that a quarter of the calls it receives every week are about eating problems. One letter in *TV Times* provoked a mailbag of 800, all from women asking for help with eating problems. Almost ninety per cent of the patients of a special clinic solely for eating disorders set up in Cincinnati in 1977 are women, and all are extremely distressed by their apparent lack of control over eating behaviour. In some cases the eating patterns they exhibit are quite deviant from the normal population, but often they are unremarkable, except for the tremendous guilt they engender.

Women's second domain is beauty and the body. And it has often been well said that the ideals of beauty set for women, and the fashion industry that every year makes new rules for the game, are both a function of man's impulse to limit women's development. Beauty gives women a certain power over men; indeed, seduction can be a woman's prime weapon. But the battle is lost before she begins, for beauty takes much maintaining, and beauty, alone of the instruments of power, wanes with age. There is the twist: by adoring the physical beauty of women, men turn women into their own jailors.

Of the 1001 people who *Which?* magazine interviewed for its *Way to Slim*, fifty-eight per cent of the women wanted to slim for cosmetic reasons, contrasted with only nineteen per cent of the men. The women who were dieting for their looks were also the least overweight. Rather than concerning themselves with their health and fitness and with encouraging an inner beauty, women have – certainly until very recently – been preoccupied with gilding their cages. They spend vast sums of money on cosmetics and clothes, on polishing, manipulating, admiring and pummelling their bodies.

For both men and women, the female body, naked or clothed, is the most potent icon of our civilisation. In our sitting-rooms we become as familiar with the world depicted on television as we are with our own, real, world. By and large women on television are uniform. They are almost invariably of 'normal' weight and shape, and slender. The average soap opera or family show portrays women who are slim and polished and usually have a supportive role – as wife or mother or nurse. In leading roles women combine head with heart, but heart – or rather, as often as not, the 'needs' of a man and the home – wins out.

For adolescent girls the message is confusing. Be bright and independent but not too independent, for the 'real' woman is a man's woman. Be seductive, but let the man be dominant. Be slender, but keep the kitchen stove bubbling and the home fires burning. And if, throughout this juggling act, the woman remains immaculate, well-groomed, then success, fame and happiness can be hers.

In Great Britain alone, over ten million images of women naked to the waist are printed every day in popular newspapers. The female body is everywhere – on billboards and magazine covers, in shop window displays, selling rum, car radios, double glazing, cheese, insurance and rust remover. As we wait for a train our eyes are forced to wander over bits of women displayed on posters – Pretty Polly legs, a Lovable body, a Colgate smile, Silvikrin hair, the Lee bottom. The images and the fantasies that go with them say: use our product, look like this, and men will pay up. Be beautiful and be bought chocolates and jewels, be wined and dined, be bedded and married and happy. Like the products her body is used to sell, woman becomes a commodity on the market. She is both bait and catch.

A woman is aware that her own body does not compare well with the bodies on the posters, which encourage her, as they do men, to see female bodies as objects. Jo Spence, a photographer who collects images of women, has observed the fragmentation techniques used by advertising agencies. In Gina Newson's film *Body Images*, made in 1981, she said:

> You get on one page a pair of lips, you turn over and there's a pair of legs; turn over and there are eyes: turn over and there's a face that's been hacked in half by the edge of the page. It turns the woman into a fetish. She's completely

ripped out of time. A little bit of her comes to represent her, in the image.

It is hard for women to see themselves whole. Neither, very often, do men see women whole. 'I'm a bum man.' 'I'm a tits man.' 'I go for legs.' Women also fix their attention, less cheerfully, on parts of their body. 'My bottom is too big.' 'My nose is all wrong and my bosom is too small.' 'My problem is my lumpy thighs.' Men and women think of women's bodies as a collection of parts. Living in an age when defective parts of machines, and now defective organs inside the human body, are pulled out, thrown away and replaced, women have a constant sense of inadequacy about the 'defective' parts of their body.

The self-hatred syndrome

Many women come to hate their bodies, and try with the help of doctors to treat their 'defective parts' literally as if they were machinery. In 1979, 300,000 American women had their breasts enlarged, usually with silicone implants; and every year between 15,000 and 20,000 American women have their breasts reduced in operations that frequently fail and leave them grossly disfigured. Barbarous methods of losing weight have now been devised. By-pass surgery to remove a portion of the intestine is usually followed by severe, prolonged and repulsive gut problems, and can kill. Stapling, an operation that closes off the upper portion of the stomach with sterilised staples, is also dangerous, and the staples are liable to tear.

Jaw-wiring has been in the news in Great Britain recently. This is a procedure which requires a woman to live on a liquid diet for a year or more, with her jaws wired shut. Any woman put on this regime will of course lose weight, and after a while she will learn how to talk, after a fashion. Cases followed up after the jaws have been unwired usually show massive and dramatic weight gain. The following report appeared in the *Sun* in January 1983:

Hairdresser Lynne Oakley, who shed 10 stone in two years, has put most of it back on again – in two months. The wires doctors put on her jaws to stop her eating snapped before Christmas – and so did her willpower. Lynne, 30, who tips the scales at 24 stone, said yesterday: 'It happened at the worst time when everybody was eating and drinking'. She was down to 15 stone when she abandoned her battle of the bulge. Now she's going to start again.

The long-term 'success' rate of jaw-wiring is not known, because it is a new technique. Probably the women who subject themselves to jaw-wiring will in time regain the weight they lost.

Most of the women who submit themselves to these procedures are grossly obese, to the point at which their lives are in danger; or their obesity prevents some other surgical operation. But in the USA some by no means obese women have found doctors willing to carry out these procedures. What causes the self-hatred that drives women to these drastic ends? It is not merely because their bodies do not conform to current standards of attractiveness. Such women have come to think of their bodies as 'things'. A young girl in Gina Newson's film says:

> I remember hearing this poem once, by Leonard Cohen. He was writing about his mother. He said 'She viewed her whole body like a scar grown over some earlier perfection'. And I knew what that meant as if I'd written it myself, I knew from my soul. There's some very nice 'me' inside and it's just spoiled by the way I look. I feel so fat and ugly.

The girl was shown in silhouette; she could not bear to be seen. Gina Newson told me that she was normal size, even on the slender side, and was in no way ugly.

For women fatness means ugliness, and to be ugly is to be rejected, lonely, on the margins of society. And so, by an appalling association of ideas, some girls and women who are lonely and feel rejected come to believe that this is because they are ugly and fat, even when by any sensible standard they are no such thing. No wonder women go on diets.

A woman is taught to think of her body as a thing

205

separate from her inner self. And yet she is also taught that her body is her means of expression. Boys are brought up to direct their energies outwards; girls are trained to project their personalities by means of physical attractiveness. In her book *Why Women Fail*, the psychiatrist Ann Dally writes about self-destruction. This, she says, is one of

the biggest handicaps that women face today. It reveals an inability to choose constructively in a world of choice or to find a positive way out of dilemmas created by choice. Even time-honoured female preoccupations such as catching a man are liable in our society to be self-destructive.

In dieting, women turn their energies in on themselves, often in fear and distress, and concentrate on the private safe world of their own body – but which then, when the diet fails, they feel has let them down too. Dieting begins as a comforting occupation which avoids conflict and engagement with the unknown, the world outside, and then becomes a new and inescapable ground on which battles are lost.

These wars start early. The young girl with anorexia nervosa uses her body both as an object of her own will and as her one means of self-expression. Abandoning interaction with her family and with the world, the anorexic girl holds tight to the only territory which she feels to be her own: her shrinking body. Some anorexics say they would rather die than give up this control. Some do die.

Although anorexia is defined as a disorder separate from dieting, many anorexics begin by dieting. And a severe diet undertaken by a girl whose normal food includes a lot of junk may induce pathological loss of appetite for biochemical reasons alone. However it may be triggered though, anorexia nervosa is not a disease but a neurosis, a severe maladaptation with a background of circumstances which are common to all women. Cases of anorexia nervosa are increasing, and are no longer confined to middle-class adolescent girls.

In her classic work *Eating Disorders: Obesity, Anorexia Nervosa and the Person Within*, Professor

Hilde Bruch outlines hundreds of case histories. Anorexics, she says, tend to be above average in intelligence, and speak lucidly about their feelings. One girl whom Professor Bruch was treating said: 'This was something I could control. I know my body can take anything.' Another, by contrast, was afraid of being strong: 'Her ideal was to be weak, ethereal and thin, so that she could accept everybody's help without feeling guilty.' For Sheila MacLeod, who has written of her own experience in *The Art of Starvation*, being plump suggested being fattened for the kill; alternatively, being swallowed up by family, school and university.

For some women, becoming thin is a bid for autonomy. The woman with developed pathological anorexia goes so far as to deny anyone access to her when they offer food, or the comfort and love associated with food. This contrasts markedly with the dieter, who wants to fit in with society's standards. Anorexics lose any real perception of body size; in their diminishing world they cannot see that they are becoming skeletal.

New eating disorders are now being identified. The latest to hit the headlines of the women's pages is bulimia. Bulimics have a normal body weight which they maintain by vomiting, as often as two or three times a day. Some women settle on this means of controlling their weight and use it for years. So too do some sportsmen who must keep their weight down – jockeys, for example. Bulimia, which is painful unless you have developed stomach muscles, eventually strips teeth of their enamel and soaks the digestive system with acid. Vomiting to avoid weight gain is a practice that the bulimic will keep secret. It isolates her, in our society, even more than the taking of illegal drugs.

A single small announcement was placed in *Cosmopolitan* asking bulimic readers to complete a questionnaire. Over 1000 replies were received. Over half this number of women made themselves vomit at least daily; about seventy per cent were generally disturbed; eighty-nine per cent had 'profoundly disturbed attitudes to food and eating'. Although most of the women felt they needed medical help, only thirty per cent had mentioned their habit to a doctor. Bulimia is not often noticed, because sufferers usually eat normally, have a normal weight, and the need for secrecy, and the sense of shame and disgust they feel, keep them underground. Magazine articles in which women talk about having been anorexic are quite common nowadays. But I have yet to read a piece about a woman saying that she throws up and is proud of it.

Women, food and society

There is something horrifyingly wrong with a society that drives women to diet constantly, to starve themselves beyond help, to void their food. These conditions are commonplace in our society.

The condition of women preoccupied with their weight is pitiable: they blame themselves, punish themselves; allow themselves to be subjected to 'aversion therapy' in which they receive an electric shock when confronted with chocolate; conditioned by slimming clubs to re-train all thoughts about food; told that their instincts to nourish and be nourished are bad.

Women are taught to be afraid of food. For dieters the fear develops because diets do not work and increase the desire for food. Many women are caught in a trap which makes food, the source of life, that which is most to be feared. No wonder that so many women have 'disordered' eating habits.

Priests and doctors have put the weight of their authority on the side of body-hatred. Within Christianity the spirit is at war with the flesh and, since the Fall, it has been woman's flesh that has tempted man into evil. The Virgin Mary, pure and beautiful and often depicted as slim, is not an exception and proves the rule – for, nlike any earthly mother, she is a virgin. In *The Second Sex* Simone de Beauvoir writes:

> The flesh that is for the Christian the hostile *other*, is woman. In her, the Christian finds incarnated the temptations of the world, the flesh and the devil. All the fathers of the church insist on the idea that she led Adam into sin.

Christianity associates woman with the earth, with the

old pre-Christian religions and so with the devil, whom Christians pictured as a perversion of the horned gods worshipped before Christianity in Europe. Women who understood the ways of the earth, knew the plants and herbs that would restore well-being, heal wounds and help in illness, were labelled witches and destroyed, and much of their knowledge with them.

In the Middle Ages and well beyond, Church and state both enforced fear and suspicion of woman's body. 'Get thee to a nunnery,' Hamlet says to Ophelia, who goes mad. Othello eventually believes that Desdemona is lustful and murders her. Chastity belts, female circumcision, convents, chaperones were all means used to protect men against the supposed carnal impulses of women, and to protect women against themselves.

Rampant suspicion of women's sexuality lay behind many so-called 'scientific' beliefs propounded by doctors in the nineteenth century. The *Journal of the American Medical Association* in 1894 recommended treating sexual desire at the menopause with hot douches of up to ten quarts daily and leeches to take fluid from the region of the uterus. The physician's conclusion sounds much like that of a modern diet doctor. 'Such patients have so much lack of confidence in themselves, their physicians and their friends, that they have not the willpower to keep up a systematic course of treatment.'

Writing in 1910, Havelock Ellis found that the belief, spread by doctors as scientific orthodoxy, that men and women breathed differently – men 'abdominally' and women 'thoracically' – stemmed from the fact that the women measured had crushed their stomachs with corsets. In *The Unfashionable Human Body*, social historian Bernard Rudofsky says: 'The physician, whose business it is to keep us in good working order, was then as reluctant to interfere with fashion's dictate as he is today.'

Jane Fonda to her cost found that Rudofsky was right when, as a model and then as a film star, she not only dieted obsessively but, to force her weight down, took drugs for over ten years.

No doctor ever told me of their side effects. No doctor

ever took the time, or showed enough interest, to ask just how and why we were using these amphetamines. Nor did any doctor warn us that we could become addicted to them – as I did.

Today, food has replaced sex as the focus of women's disgust and guilt. It is fatness that leads to damnation: slimness through dieting is the salvation.

The dos and don'ts of the diet books are the new dogma, the lists of forbidden and allowed foods the new catechism; and the diet doctor replaces the priest and physician of the past as woman's guide to grace. When organised religion is absent other rituals take its place. It is no accident that dieting is most widespread and diet doctors most powerful in those countries, mostly Protestant, where religion has lost its grip. And, just as Christians are taught that their bodies are vessels of sin and that salvation is through faith, so dieters can come to believe that their struggles and their failures only prove the need constantly to discipline and punish the body.

The futility of dieting fuels some women's sense of worthlessness. Others diet because they feel that as long as they are fat – in their own eyes – their life has not started, and that dieting will solve their problems. 'When I am thin, then . . .' – I will be beautiful, or healthy, or lovable, or happy, or successful, or effective. The *Which? Way to Slim* gives sober counsel to its readers:

> Losing weight will not of itself guarantee that you will find a marriage partner or improve your relationship with the one you have. You should regard your slimming as a rational task which will result in weight loss – not as a magic solution to all your ills.

The fragile ideal

Has woman's flesh always been despised? By no means. The image of the Earth Mother has its origins in agriculture. It was women, there is little doubt, who first tilled the soil, planted, sowed and cultivated the earth, and gathered in the harvest. When settled communities began to be established, it was the women with flesh who were best protected against times of famine, most healthy, and most likely to bear healthy children. Fertility symbols often take the form of depictions of hugely fat women.

The connection between beauty and the promise of fertility and fecundity has been made for centuries in art. The paintings of Rubens and Rembrandt, and later of Courbet and Renoir, all celebrate the abundance of female flesh and a voluptuous sexuality.

In Europe, slenderness in women was first desired in the eighteenth century. In the Age of Enlightenment, the emerging middle classes had less fear of disease, plague and famine were no longer rampant, and the food supply was more assured. Man required a companion on his now extended journey through life.

The woman of leisure came to be associated with the finer things of life: with art and literature, taste and refinement. Sense and sensibility were the hallmarks of an ideal marriage partner. The wife of the peasant continued to be buxom; the wife of the gentleman was sensitive, her elegantly slender body betraying little sign of the basic functions of life, her soft white hands giving no sign of work, her delicate complexion unmarked by weather. That, at any rate, was the image, the ideal, of female slenderness.

As the concept of companionship implies, women were being raised from an entirely subordinate role to one of greater equality, one more 'like men'. And, of course, the male physique – translated to a woman's body – is slim. In her book *Fat and Thin*, medical historian Anne Scott Beller says:

> People tend to ape their betters, and women's aspirations to the unmodulated physiques of men express unvoiced, and until recently probably largely unconscious, judgements about the nature of male status and privilege compared with their own.

The *grandes dames* of the Parisian *salons*, famous for their wit, charm and intelligence, had posed a certain threat to men. Thereafter, the second image of the ideal female shape did not so much develop out of the first as parody it.

The nineteenth-century lady was fragile and languorous, liable to fainting fits and to the vapours. Her vulnerability emphasised the strength, power and superiority of the man. The pallor of a Dame aux Camélias was a sign of a deadly all-too delicate constitution. Consumption became chic. This ethereal creature did not so much diet as starve herself. She was too unworldly for such coarse matters as food. She took enemas and purgatives to maintain her tiny waist. Her tightly laced corsets made sure she could not digest food properly when she did eat. Her body weak and crushed, she often miscarried. That, at any rate, was the image to which so many Victorian women were expected to aspire, and their failure, as their bodies resisted their regimes, must have made them as guilty and ashamed as any female dieter today.

In *Illness as Metaphor* Susan Sontag says:

> Twentieth-century women's fashions (with their cult of thinness) are the last stronghold of the metaphors associated with the romanticising of TB in the late eighteenth and early nineteenth centuries.

Independence or vulnerability

Since the early 1960s – years in which the contraceptive Pill has removed the risk of pregnancy from sex, and the women's movement has grown – dieting has engulfed the women of the West. In some respects the compulsion to diet is similar to the contrasting forces behind the ideals of slimness prevailing in the eighteenth and nineteenth centuries. Today, some women diet to assert their sexual freedom, seeing the sexually active body as lean, smooth and honed. Others, by contrast, diet to show an appealing vulnerability, seeing the submissive body as slim, soft and petted. These opposing ideals can resonate against each other, causing new confusions. An unpleasant recent example is the rise of the child model and movie star, the adolescent bodies of Brooke Shields and Jodie Foster becoming sex symbols in *Pretty Baby* and *Taxi Driver*.

Women's bodies, or rather the images of ideal women's

bodies, are on show everywhere. Ever since Twiggy's astounding success as a model in Great Britain and the USA, millions of women have half starved themselves in futile attempts to achieve her figure.

Attractive women are seen as young and slim, and therefore many older women have found themselves neglected, rejected and abandoned by their husbands – traded in for a younger model. Many such women, preferring to lose their dignity rather than their man, have starved themselves into scrawny versions of their post-adolescent rivals. Hilde Bruch comments:

> It is impossible to assess the cost in serenity, relaxation and efficiency of this abnormal, overslim fashionable appearance. It produces serious psychological tensions to feel compelled to be thinner than one's natural make-up and style of living demand. I do not know how often people are aware of the emotional sacrifice of staying slim.

As time passes women very often find that, unless they exercise, the only way they can stay slim is to submit to a state of perpetual semi-starvation, perhaps also to take drugs, and are quite likely to form extremely disordered eating patterns. The consequence is depression, exhaustion and illness, and a reduced life expectancy. In these circumstances it is better to fail. Professor Bruch continues:

> There is a great deal of talk about the weakness and self indulgence of overweight people who eat 'too much'. Very little is said about the selfishness and self indulgence involved in a life which makes one's appearance the centre of all values.

We all need a sense of control over ourselves and our lives. But we have lost a sense of control, restraint, mastery. Anything goes; the bomb may drop; redundancy is round the corner. The woman who chooses not to restrain her sexual appetite is likely to transfer her need for some form of restraint on to food. Other women diet just in order to be able to hold some sense of order. The language women dieters use to describe their fears is significant. 'I mustn't let myself go.' 'I'm afraid of my fat taking me over.' 'My body's out of control.' 'I feel helpless when I gain weight.' The rituals of the diet regimes, with their lists and numbers and orders of the day, are a sure sign of a general malaise. The sad irony is that dieting itself creates the alienation from the body, the weakness, illness and flabbiness that the dieter most fears. Dieting is now the most widespread self-destructive activity known to woman.

Mastery is a male concept. The women most concerned to prove themselves the equal of men, in men's domains such as business and industry, are particularly likely to see pencil thinness as the sign of dynamism, mind over matter, and a rigid armour typical of the male executive. The image is not that of an earthy siren – a Dorothy Lamour, Marilyn Monroe or Sophia Loren – but of heady adventuresses such as Bette Davis, Joan Crawford and Katharine Hepburn, mannish, independent and tough.

Other women try to make sense of the demands put on them, and the demand they put on themselves, to be both independent and also good wives, lovers and mothers, to work well in the office and at home, to satisfy colleagues, man and children. Such women too are liable to be driven into themselves and seek control by dieting, just as much as the adolescent.

Dieting is liable to be an attempt to compensate for the lack of control women feel over their lives. Women from all walks of life and all classes feel confused because of conflicting desires to be mother, home-maker and also independent people with their own lives, and are liable to retreat into the one area they think they can control: their bodies. Sadly, defeat in dieting is likely to be the most inevitable defeat of all.

The swings from self-denial to self-indulgence, from fasting to feasting – all of which may involve secret or furtive eating – reflect woman's oscillation between her conflicting roles. For the younger woman the pressure is more than ever to be thin. The Superwoman image cultivated by Helen Gurley Brown of *Cosmopolitan* and by Shirley Conran in Great Britain is an image of both femininity and independence: these women represent themselves as having it all ways. 'If only I could look like that,' other women think, go on another diet, and fail again – and again.

Self-doubt, anxiety, lack of confidence, confusion, self-destructiveness: these are emotions most women know all too well. Successful women too: 'Will I be lovable if I'm strong and independent?' 'Will my children hate me for having a career?' 'If I choose to stay at home and care for my family will I regret it later?' Women's magazines are full of questions like these.

Women are now becoming more free not only in their minds but in their bodies also – with much hesitation. The realisation is dawning that dieting is a lonely and frustrating business that usually fails; and also that the rules of the calorie charts, the instructions of the diet doctors, the obedience and submission involved in dieting, the fragility and weakness that come with loss of weight, are all repulsive as well as futile.

As they turn away from spending their lives being told what to do, women should also turn away from the regulations and restrictions and, yes, the persecution of dieting regimes and diet doctors. Men are more and more discovering the value of their emotional selves. Women have the opportunity to discover the strength and power of their physical selves.

This does not mean opting for the Earth Mother image, which is just as limiting as the Slender Superwoman stereotype. But it is time to abandon the notion that a woman needs to be – should be – thin to be the best or proper kind of woman. It is time that this adolescent image is seen for what it is, and for women to find out what is the best shape and size for themselves as individuals. It is time, too, to abandon the costly and futile wars that women fight against their own bodies, to abandon the diet regimes that weaken them, depress them, and eventually – ironically – make them fat.

It is time for women to get on the move.

CHAPTER SEVEN

The Active Woman

> It is vain to say human beings ought to be satisfied with
> tranquillity: they must have action, and they will make it if
> they cannot find it. Millions are condemned to a stiller fate
> than mine, and millions are in silent revolt against their lot.
> Women are supposed to be very calm generally; but
> women feel just as men feel; they need exercise for their
> faculties and a field for their efforts as much as their
> brothers do; they suffer from too rigid a constraint, too
> absolute a stagnation, precisely as men suffer.
> CHARLOTTE BRONTË
> *Jane Eyre*

> What is now called the nature of women is an eminently
> artificial thing, the result of forced repressing in some
> directions, unnatural stimulation in others. It may be
> asserted without scruple, that no other class of dependants
> have had their character so entirely distorted from its
> natural proportions.
> JOHN STUART MILL
> *The Subjection of Women*

Finding yourself

For women exercise is a sure way to self-discovery and
self-realisation. Accustomed to see themselves, and be
seen, as passive objects, many women find the effects of
exercise a revelation. Interviewed in San Luis Obispo,
California, for *Running* magazine, Alice Werbel spoke of
her first running steps, age fifty-seven, and after her
husband Ernie had retired:

Your children are gone; you must get up and do something. We started to take long walks. We walked by the High School track, and one day I said – why don't we run, just a quarter mile or so? Then one day, we got to run a mile.

That was in 1973. The first race Alice entered was the 10,000 metre run at the Senior Olympics held at Irvine. Her son had sent her a wool warm-up suit and, knowing no better, she ran the race under the Californian summer sun wearing it. Afterwards she was told that her time of fifty-three minutes was a world record for women aged between fifty-five and sixty. In 1981 she held six world records, for distances between 800 metres and the one-hour run. In 1983, at the age of sixty-eight, she said: 'I so often wish that people could understand that they had it within them. You feel sometimes that you shouldn't be out there training on the track; that you should be in a rocking chair.'

At eight in the morning on Sunday 29 March 1981 Sue Goggin, a forty-year-old mother of three, was at the gates of Greenwich Park to watch the start of the first London marathon. 'Oh what admiration I had for all those people, especially the old. If they can do it, so can I at forty,' she wrote. She started to jog – finding at first that she couldn't run fast enough to catch the bus to work. Then she joined the *London 1982/50* group, training to complete the second London marathon, on Sunday 9 May 1982; which she did, in a time of four hours fifty-seven minutes. For her, running has given her a new freedom: 'It is marvellous to shut the front door and leave all the hubbub and squabbles of three children behind – let Dad sort it out for a while, and feel the freedom of running with one's own thoughts.'

Helen Johnston, a woman of twenty-eight, was part of the same London marathon team; she finished in four hours twenty-one minutes. For her, changed shape, not weight, was a benefit of running:

My weight has stayed much the same, although I eat more. Running makes me so hungry! A lot of women complain about flabby thighs. Mine used to be, but running has firmed them up – also backside. I just feel so healthy and fit!

217

Helen also found just how much many men need to believe that women are and should be passive creatures, objects of admiration but not active, energetic and strong. She was the victim not only of verbal sexual aggression from men as she passed by on the run but also of threatened physical aggression.

> Most scary are the kerb crawlers. I have nightmares of being dragged into the car. Then there are the pedestrians. The men are the most threatening and the most crude. All this upsets me, makes me angry, and sometimes I have honestly been very frightened.

When she started to run, Helen did not know how to handle this kind of bad experience. But once her body was in training she answered back.

Calm and zest

Women report various benefits from exercise: sleep becomes deeper, period pains subside, they feel calmer and gain zest. Lucilla Deane, another young member of the London marathon team, said:

> Physically I just felt more alive. I've always been rather a bad sleeper and suddenly I find, now, that I go out like a light. I felt that my body was using its food more efficiently. I don't feel hungry for at least an hour or two after a run. What I do eat I feel is being metabolised more efficiently now.

Some psychologists in the USA are discovering the effectiveness of exercise compared with conventional psychoanalytical methods in raising personal awareness and dealing with anxiety and depression. In her book *Women and Sports*, Janice Kaplan describes the work of Dyveke Spino, once a clinical psychologist and now an Olympic coach, who uses physical activity in her work with groups of women. Referring to the Greek ideal of the integration of mind, body and spirit she says: 'You can't deal with the mind and emotions unless you pay attention to sports and games.'

Using movement therapy and jogging and running, she encourages women to get in touch with an energy they were unaware they had and to find an untapped inner strength and vitality: 'Most women have a lot of self-doubt and built-in masochism. They don't really know themselves, and don't know how to go into the world and grab what they want.'

A run can be just as effective a therapy for depression as a session on the couch. An American psychologist, interested in the benefits of jogging, gave one group of people conventional analysis for an hour, one by one; and took a second group out together for half an hour's run. The joggers showed more improvement in their general sense of well-being and control over their lives; and they saved a lot of money, too.

To own one's body

I began to jog, and then run, almost a decade after I became a student. I didn't choose to because of thinking that it is the only suitable form of exercise; it isn't. But it is simple and convenient. In Great Britain you can run almost anywhere, almost any time, and it's cheap: all you need is a T-shirt, a pair of shorts, running shoes, and a tracksuit for warming up and for cold weather.

For me the sensation of moving swiftly through the air unhampered by the usual layers of clothing, handbags and high heels, was extraordinary. On my first runs, just of ten and then twenty minutes, I felt the flush of warmth through my body as my sluggish circulation started to work hard; and, afterwards, heaving lungs, tingling skin, the glow of physical exertion and, later, the beginnings of real hunger. These sensations, I came to realise, with a pang, are those of childhood. A long time before, and I didn't know when, I had put them aside, along with tree-climbing and make-believe.

Mobility is crucial to the growth process of children; it is the key to their sense of themselves in the world. We cannot know much about our bodies unless we move them; and this is why children are constantly on the move, touching and exploring the space around them and their place within it. Neurologist Paul Schilder's work has shown him that when children stop moving they stop learning. This has special significance for the overweight and the obese. Commenting on Schilder's work in her book *Eating Disorders*, Professor Hilde Bruch writes, 'The inactivity so characteristic of obese people thus appears to be related to their often disturbed body concept.'

She is suggesting that some people become obese in part because of inactivity and, moreover, that inactivity is sometimes pathological, springing from fear of the world and fear of learning. Obese people often report feelings of alienation from their bodies; and their supposed calm and contentment may come from a sense of powerlessness and anxiety about being active. Some obese people, women in particular, need a lot of encouragement to follow an exercise programme.

In the first months of running I made several other discoveries. My skin gained a bloom and a glow. Quite soon I stopped puffing and gasping, as my body adapted to the new stresses I put on it. I felt that my lungs were expanding, learning a new rhythm of inhalation and exhalation which soothed me as I ran. Without becoming bulky my muscles started to become more defined and smoother, and my hair grew thicker and glossier.

I gained respect for my body, which I had so often distrusted and despised. I had no intention – nor have I now – of running races, let alone marathons; for me, running was and is for health and well-being. So as one running companion pushed me to run faster and longer, I moaned and complained: I was convinced that I couldn't do it, that I didn't want to do it, that it was too much for me. I resisted achievement with every technique. He was unimpressed; and to my surprise and – I must admit – pleasure, I found I could do it!

At school and university words were my means of expression; I avoided games at school, I am a poor and fearful swimmer and never learnt to play tennis. Sport was something sporty people did, so I was rather embarrassed to discover that I loved the experience and the effects of running. The world of physical expression is not one in which you can be smarter or cleverer; words don't come into it. It became a new way of being for me which I found exciting, liberating, and so a little dangerous and scary.

I began to test my new reliable body on runs of first two,

220

then three, then four and a half miles. It no longer mattered that I thought my body was an odd shape; for I was enjoying it, being in my body rather than looking at it from the outside. For the first time since childhood, I had the sense that I owned my body.

Having run three or four times a week for a few months, I found a real and reliable sense of hunger. In the mornings I looked forward to my breakfast – muesli and yoghurt and a pot of tea – but no longer needed to have lunch just because it was 'lunchtime'. I eat when I'm hungry. My appetite for starchy foods increased spontaneously, which at first worried me. But I now know that the active body needs a lot of whole, unprocessed, cereals and vegetables. At the same time my appetite for meat, sweets, chocolate, alcohol and cigarettes decreased. I still eat cakes and have a drink from time to time, and the occasional cigarette; but I no longer treat myself to a pudding as a way of trying to calm some general sense of dissatisfaction.

I put on weight: about six pounds. The old part of me was horrified! But I was pleased with my body, and people kept telling me how slim I was: the catch-all compliment which often really means 'How well you look'. Loath to part with old habits, I sometimes deprived myself of food, but then I came to acknowledge that the extra pounds belong to me, are part of my body as I feel it should be. And I recognised, and it was a shock, that what I used to label my neuroses – anxiety, depression, listlessness, hopelessness – were at least in part caused by years of malnourishment and under-nourishment. Angst is romantic, semi-starvation is not.

In any case, I was becoming pleased with the way I looked. My body composition changed as I lost some fat and gained some heavier lean tissue.

I started to enjoy listening to my body. For a while a series of malaises and infections made me feel as if running were in some way literally jogging poisons in my body to the surface. Whatever their cause, these illnesses ceased. Yoga classes, which I had previously put off when I believed I had something 'better to do', became top priority; a couple of hours of stretching in a gym or an hour of running was never time wasted or lost, and gave me more energy and zest for my work. And I slept better.

When I started to exercise in the open air it was not just the exhilaration of being energetic that spurred me on but also the forgotten joy of being part of the physical reality of nature. I had not realised just how much time I spent looking at the world through screens: windows; books, television, film; coats, hats and mufflers.

To run free with minimum clothing is a marvellous freedom. The world I got to know was that of Kensington Gardens and Hyde Park. I felt the different textures underfoot; tarmac, gravel, grass firm and muddy, snow. I watched the park grow as spring became summer, in different light and different weather. Wind and rain were simply that – cold and wet against the skin, bracing, not something to huddle up against. I felt the seasons change as shoots appeared, then leaves emerged emerald green, then darker in summer, then brown and gold in the autumn. I was within my own experience, as I passed by and came to know the people with their dogs, other runners whose route was clockwise, the tramp whose territory is a particular bench by the Royal Garden Hotel, the old lady forever painting the ornamental garden by Kensington Palace, from the east side of the vine arbour.

Exercising the body is a positive discipline, in contrast with the negative discipline of dieting. Any normal person on a diet longs for it to end. But once the body has become accustomed to exercise, a run, a dance session, a yoga class is something to look forward to: a freedom, not a restriction.

It all sounds simple and inviting. As Alice Werbel found, it is just a matter of being like a child again – getting up and running, or swimming, or dancing, for fun. But in practice, for women there are more complex issues; Helen Johnston experienced one. And there are others: taboos, self-doubt, family, social demands, prejudice, inhibitions, prohibitions.

Losing and winning

Women's attitudes towards sport influences their attitudes to exercise and physical activity. As they grow up, girls are encouraged to be more sedentary than boys. The very word 'tomboy' used, affectionately or not, of a girl nearing puberty speaks worlds.

Again and again girls and women are prevented from participating in sports regarded as men's domain. In Great Britain, the Equal Opportunities Commission championed the case of Theresa Bennett, whom the Football Association had prohibited from playing in an under-twelve league. She won her case, but lost it on appeal. Evidence was put forward on Theresa's behalf that she was pre-pubertal and a 'guided missile in football boots'. Lord Denning set these pleas aside and refused further appeals, finally saying, 'We don't enquire about the age of ladies.'

Elizabeth Ferris, a doctor specialising in sports medicine, won the Bronze medal for diving in the Rome Olympics in 1960. At school her headmistress had her examined by a cardiologist on the grounds that so much training must be bad for a girl's heart. A less determined girl would have been discouraged. Kathrine Switzer is public relations director of Avon Products Inc. responsible for their involvement in women's running. In 1967 she entered the Boston marathon, purportedly an 'open' event, as 'K Switzer', knowing that race officials would otherwise cancel her entry. In the event it took a hefty shoulder-charge from her boy-friend to prevent a race marshal manhandling her out of the race, which she completed.

And it was not so long ago that award-winning football writer Brian Glanville of the *Sunday Times* made it clear that in his view sport was all right for ladies but questionable for women: 'There is no reason why a woman should not indulge in any kind of sport she wishes.' (It's difficult to imagine a writer saying: 'There is no reason why a man should not indulge in any kind of sport he wishes.') Glanville goes on:

> A girl who goes out to run, swim, or play tennis for the joy of it is still being a girl. But a girl who slogs away all winter in a gymnasium lifting weights so she can beat other girls in the summer is behaving like an imitation man.

Winning is all right for boys. But a girl who wants to win

– or even to exert herself to her utmost – is questioned. Rejecting a proposal that a woman's 3000-metre race should be included in the 1980 Games the International Olympic Committee said that it was 'a little too strenuous'.

No wonder that a recent survey in Great Britain showed that only forty per cent of girls play any sports outside school and that half intend to give up all sport after leaving school. In contrast seventy per cent of boys played sport outside school and only twenty per cent intended to give up sport after school. The boys had been encouraged; the girls had been discouraged.

The image of the Olympic Games is the summit of athletic ability and the manifestation of the true spirit of sport, where to win is not so glorious as to take part. But Baron Pierre de Coubertin, founder of the modern Olympic movement, fought successfully to keep women out of the Games. Women's track and field events were organised separately from the Olympics in the early years of this century. The first women's international meeting took place in Monte Carlo in 1921: over 100 women from five countries took part. The next year 300 competitors from seven countries participated, and it was decided to form a Women's World Olympics. After pressure from the Olympic Games organisers the name was changed to the Women's World Games. These were held in 1922 in Paris. Men's track events such as the 400 and 1500 metres were reduced to 300 and 1000 metres. For the second Women's World Games in 1926, in Sweden, ten countries were represented in thirteen events. In his book *Catching Up the Men*, Ken Dyer observed that at this point women's athletics 'had grown from almost nothing to a major force on the sporting scene, with a programme almost as varied as men's and approaching theirs in level of participant support'. Only then was the perennial request that women be allowed to compete in the Olympic Games grudgingly accepted, for the 1928 Games. There were two conditions: women were only admitted provisionally and were confined to five events.

The all-male Olympic Committee thus effectively restricted what was becoming a flourishing and vigorous development. In the 1928 Games, held in Amsterdam, the

800-metre world record for women was broken by Lina Radke. As she and other competitors crossed the line, they collapsed from exhaustion. As a result the administrators banned all women's track races except the 100 metres, and thereafter the inclusion of every woman's track event had to be fought for. The 800-metre track event only reappeared in 1960, the year in which Elizabeth Ferris competed as a diver. Addressing a congress on women and sport in Rome twenty years later Dr Ferris said:

> Even in 1960 only 600 of the 5,000 odd competitors were women, and they only competed in 6 of the 17 sports. We women, inside our very separate compound in the Olympic village, were savagely protected by patrolling guards who paced, panther-like, up and down outside a wire fence that was so high that not even the gold-medallist in the pole-vault could have got over it.

The women's 200-metre race was added in 1948, the 400 metres in 1964 and the 1500 metres in 1972.

The hardest struggle for women has been to gain acceptance for long-distance running events in the Olympics. It is only in 1984 that the 3000 metres and the marathon have been included. The absurdity of these delays is emphasised by the fact that it is in endurance events that womens' achievements are the greatest. Ann Sayer recently took the all-comers' record for the 840-mile Lands End to John O'Groats walk, beating the previous record set by a man. (Asked how she managed to finish in thirteen days she said that she could only take two weeks off from work and had to be in the office the next day.) The American Penny Lee Dean holds the England to France cross-channel swimming record. Canadian Cynthia Nicholas holds the two-way cross-channel record. In 1980 Naomi James held the solo round-the-world sailing record. In long-distance, endurance events women have less upper body strength than men but compensate with comparable leg strength. And there is good evidence that in long-distance events women can regulate their body temperature better than men, and also that they use body fat as fuel more efficiently.

Avery Brundage, President of the International

Olympics Committee from 1952 to 1972, was, in power and long service, to the Olympics movement what J Edgar Hoover was to American law enforcement. Brundage always made it clear that he, like any Victorian, was interested in ladies, not in women, in sport. He once said, 'I am fed up to the ears with women as track and field competitors. As swimmers and divers girls are beautiful and adroit as they are ineffective and unpleasing on the track.'

Discouraged at school, women are given inferior facilities at all levels. The 1981 – 82 allocation for the University of London Rowing Club was £7000. The club has a man's team and a woman's team, with equal numbers in each: £200 was allocated to the women's team. In all professional sports, prizes for women professionals are far lower than those for men. But when they persevere and endure the training that makes champions, women are told they are 'unfeminine'. The great long-distance running coach Percy Cerutty had this to say: 'Who wants straight-legged, narrow-hipped, big-shouldered, powerful women, aggressive and ferocious in physique and attitude?' Clearly such a woman would be more than Percy could handle!

Women are catching up

Common sense suggests that women have in certain respects powers of endurance superior to those of men: women's bodies are built to bear children. Miki Gorman was the first woman home in the Boston marathon twice, in 1974 and 1977, having her first baby at the age of forty in between. 'Compared with having a baby, a marathon is easy,' she said. And during the 1970s, while the men's world record for the marathon remained at the 2.08.33 set by Derek Clayton, the women's world record was broken sixteen times, falling from 3.02.53 to 2.27.33. (In 1984 the records stood at Alberto Salazar's 2.08.13 and Joan Benoit's 2.22.42).

Why, then, did it take until the 1984 Games for the women's marathon to be accepted as an Olympic event? Elizabeth Ferris asked this question of a woman associate of the International Olympic Committee before the 1980 Moscow Games, at a time when thousands of women were competing in long-distance races. Eventually the reason given, said Dr Ferris, was that:

> She had seen a woman cross-country skier vomit at the end of a race, and this had offended her dreadfully. No woman, in her opinion, should be so exposed and vulnerable – it was against all her deeply embedded views about what it means to be a woman.

It is not only men's attitudes to women in sports that have held women back. Women, too, have resisted achievement. In Great Britain this attitude began to change dramatically in 1981. The staggering increase in interest in long-distance running triggered by the first London marathon in 1981 disguised an even more extraordinary commitment from women.

In 1978, according to statistics compiled by veteran runner John Walsh, just 1789 British people completed a marathon; of these, a mere forty-eight were women. In 1979 and 1980 Walsh kept records only of those who finished in a time of less than four hours; the ratio of women to men remained under one in thirty. By contrast, of the 17,906 runners who registered for the 1982 London marathon, 1363 were women. Women are beginning to catch up; and women in Great Britain are catching up with a movement that started in the USA five years earlier.

The movement for fitness through sport is also becoming a movement for health through exercise. Early in 1982 co-author Geoffrey Cannon invited people with no previous experience of running to train for five months with the goal of completing the two and a half mile *Sunday Times* National Fun Run. (This *Fun Runner '82* project is described in Chapter 5, 'More Air! More Air!'). *Running* magazine, in which the invitation was carried, has a readership of ninety-three per cent men to seven per cent women. Yet more than half of the 130 replies were from women. One said: 'I desperately want to feel fit, healthy and mentally liberated from my two very adorable but demanding children. I would also very much welcome a challenge of this kind. Please be my savour!' Another replied, simply: 'My ambition is to become fit and healthy.'

After three months of jogging, thirty-eight Fun Runners were asked if regular exercise had affected their mood: were they more, or less, anxious or depressed, from time to time? This question affected the women very much more than the men. Of the thirty-eight, twenty-one said that regular exercise had definitely improved their state of mind. How much difference? This is how they replied:

Bad mood, anxiety, depression	April	July
Every day	–	–
Most days	8	–
Most weeks	5	3
Occasionally	8	10
Hardly ever/Never	–	8

I doubt that psychoanalysis would have such an effect so soon. And in July one Fun Runner decided that she would stop seeing the psychiatrist who had been treating her for some time – simply because she felt fine.

The well-being that comes from running and from other aerobic exercise takes different forms. The good effects of fresh whole food and of exercise are so simple, and yet so often they are profound. To my mind, the reason above all others for the astonishing rise in the numbers of women who now are physically active is not just the desire to get fit, stave off heart attacks or middle-age spread, or cure depression – although these are reasons, and good ones. The desire for action is the desire to rediscover the simple joy of being fully alive. The upsurge of running and dance is an appropriate reaction to our otherwise automated and sedentary lives.

'Energy is the power that drives every human being. It is not lost by exercise but maintained by it,' said Germaine Greer in *The Female Eunuch*. Ten years later Jane Fonda put Germaine Greer's thoughts into action, and the feelings of a new generation of women into words, in her *Workout Book*, saying:

I do not claim that a strong, healthy woman is automatically going to be a progressive, decent sort of person. Obviously other factors are involved in that. But I am sure that one's innate intelligence and instinct for good can be enhanced through fitness.

Watching others transform their lives through exercise, women sometimes say, or think: it must be too late for me. The slinky goddesses on television putting aerobics classes through their paces can be a discouraging sight. But even at the highest levels of achievement women are discovering that age is not a barrier to performance. Joyce Smith holds the British women's marathon record and was seen on television by millions, finishing ahead of the other women runners in the London marathon in 1981 and again in 1982 – when she was forty-four years old. Beryl Burton, the long-distance cycling champion, continued to challenge male rivals well into her forties. Mary Peters won the Olympic Pentathlon in Munich when she was thirty-three. Miki Gorman continues to set world and American records for her age in the marathon. And for an older generation, the example of Alice Werbel, who started to jog when she was fifty-seven, can be an inspiration.

The time when her children grow up and leave home can be the time of a woman's life when she can use her experience and resourcefulness to discover a new taste for adventure, with an energy and steadfastness that many a young woman may envy.

It sounds simple. In some respects it is. Any able-bodied woman can get up and go running, or swimming, or dancing. But in ways that don't directly affect men, the progress of women is dogged by taboos, self-doubt, and inhibitions. It's not only the women athletes who have a hard time.

Exercise and 'being a woman'

We adapt to the roles expected of us very early in life. Little children playing at mummies and daddies will act out the mother at home, washing-up, cooking, looking after the family; the father at the office being important, playing football with his mates at the weekend. Many television advertisements are versions of this game. No manufacturer ever sold a packet of soapflakes by showing the man of the house exclaiming with wonder at the whiteness of his wife's shorts as he fishes them out of the washer. Men are meant to be strong and independent; women are meant to be gentle and dependent: we are all taught that. A woman playing serious strenuous sport is as threatening as is a top woman executive; both women and men view such a woman as a challenge to the conventions of manliness and womanliness by which we live and limit our lives.

The sheer achievement of women tennis players, and their professionals' successful fight for prizes in line with men, has in some respects freed tennis from the pressures that discourage and inhibit women in other sports. Girls can look up to Chris Lloyd and Martina Navratilova as supreme athletes, fiercely competitive, and now possessed of some of the glamour once reserved for ballet stars.

In tennis, golf and in other sports, though, the media give more attention to the good-looking woman who is not in the top flight. Stories are printed and rumours circulate about affairs, including homosexual affairs, involving women players, but not men; and it's all right for men players to be temperamental, short of John McEnroe, but the most protest women are allowed is a squawk. A top male player is seen as attractive and admirable, and outrageous characters such as Jimmy Connors and Ilie Nastase are portrayed as lovable. But a top woman player – she's seen as a little bit strange; she is regarded with awe but also with some suspicion. She makes men, and other women, feel uncomfortable.

From time to time newspapers publish a story about a jogger who died of a heart attack, or, as a variation, about the jogger who was struck by lightning. Joggers have indeed been struck by lightning, but very rarely, and someone with a heart condition can, but also rarely, bring on a heart attack while running, although violent exercise such as squash is much more risky for someone with an undiagnosed heart condition. Readers still want to be told that jogging is bad for you; so the stories about people who die of heart attacks while sprinting for the bus, or in the midst of an unusually passionate enbrace, go unreported.

Similarly, from time to time newspapers publish a story that women runners are liable to suffer from amenorrhoea (that is to say, their periods stop). Horror! The implication is that the woman loses her fundamental womanliness because of her sport. The message of this story is like the often told accounts of those tall high-jumpers and bulky hurdlers, usually from behind the Iron Curtain, who when tested turn out by some criteria to be male, not female. On the one hand, becoming athletic is liable to render a woman neuter; on the other hand, some women athletes are men anyway.

Amenorrhoea is a common condition, as often as not caused by stress. It is perfectly true that a woman who trains very hard, running more than fifty to sixty miles a week say, may find that her periods stop or become irregular, particularly if she is thin. The condition may be reversed by taking vitamin C and iron tablets, which are in any case advisable if she eats any amount of junk food and processed sugar. But there is no evidence whatever that amenorrhoea induced by very heavy training continues after the training is eased off. Why should it? Any woman runner who regards periods as a curse can see exercise-induced amenorrhoea as a blessing. Characteristically, though, the suggestion behind the newspaper stories is: don't jog, or you may not be able to have babies – a nonsense. Exercise does not turn women into men, and it does not turn women neuter.

The beauty of strength

After starting to jog, I spent time worrying that I would develop bulging muscles – just like a man. Again, it is true that some female field athletes and body-builders develop musculature like that of men, but only if they take anabolic steroids – illegal drugs that contain male growth hormones. Without drugs, not even women weight-lifters develop bulging muscles. I had allowed myself to be inhibited by a myth; I did not do what was obvious – look at the women athletes to be seen any week on television.

It is also true that exercise sheds fat and adds lean tissue, including muscle, to a woman's body. In action, the body of a woman who takes regular exercise is clearly toned; the shape of her muscle is unobtrusive, but it shows. Here a change in what is meant by beauty in a woman is taking place – and needs to take place. Exercise creates strength, and many men other than Percy Cerutty are made to feel nervous by women who gain physical strength. But, as women find just how good they feel about themselves after exercise, they discover an inner beauty which isn't painted on. Ken Dyer ˉcites an interview with Anna Thornhill, an artist who is also a long-distance runner. She said:

> I don't worry about fitting in a fashion-type image any more. After running a marathon, and then a 7-mile race the next day and feeling no pains at all, I looked in the mirror and said, 'Body, you're okay. You're doing your job.'

And Ms Thornhill also referred to another issue that women face. What will my man think of the way I look?

> My husband doesn't want me to become too thin but I no longer want to surrender to someone else's view of sexuality; for me, functionalism and sexuality are fused. My sexuality isn't affected by the way I look any more, but by how I feel: healthy, confident and functional.

Women, and men too, are finding out that a notion of beauty that depends on a softness which is a sign of weak and unhealthy fatness is not a notion of beauty worth holding; and that the firmness of the body and the inner glow that comes with exercise are more attractive and lasting.

Some women are put off exercise because they half-believe it will make them less of a woman. Others are afraid to exercise in public, either in a dance studio or in the open air, because they are only too well aware that they don't have the body beautiful of women in advertisements. Indeed, many women are afraid to show their body in private; sexual prudery often has little to do with morals, much more to do with fear of what the other person will think of the unclothed body. Privately, women often hug thoughts that they are ugly or clumsy, even deformed.

232

Having summoned up courage to join in a jogging group or an exercise class, one of a woman's first freedoms is to find that nobody looks like the women in the rum advertisements or the magazine fashion pictures. This is for the simple reason that these models, aside from having unusual shapes and exercising daily as most models now do, are also made up and lit and photographed from special angles, all to achieve an ideal effect which is not real. Stereotypes created by the camera, just as much as by the painter, do not exist in the flesh: meet a woman who is a model, and as likely as not her most attractive feature will be one regarded as a fault by fashion and so hidden in her pictures.

An exercise class gives a woman a chance to face her fantasies, including her own horrid fantasies about her own body, and realise that everybody looks different and that beauty is in the differences, not the similarities.

The second freedom for the woman who, at whatever age, starts to exercise regularly is that some of her features she dislikes and tries to disguise – dull complexion, flabby flesh, lumpy thighs – are liable to change, sometimes quite quickly, sometimes gradually. She begins to discover the natural shape of her body, a shape which, with exercise, she will begin to appreciate in new ways.

Physical exercise is not a panacea. It is hard work, and that is why the sense of well-being that comes from exercise is lasting: it is earned. People now are moving away from the idea of beauty that implies passivity, an idea that is a hangover from Victorian days. Slimness which depends on make-up, pills and diets has nothing to do with fitness or with health. As they enjoy the inner glow that comes from exercise, women today are contradicting the notion that beauty is only skin-deep. Diets treat the body as alien, as an enemy of the mind. Exercise treats the body as integral to us, as bound up with the mind and the spirit. After three months of jogging, Kathleen Herold, a thirty-eight-year-old member of the *Fun Runner '82* group, wrote:

If I don't run every day my body lets me know that something is missing. I have lost weight, my blood pressure is down and my resting heart rate has lowered. Physically I am in better shape than I was 20 years ago; now I can run over two miles a day.

And Brenda Green, aged fifty-two:

> If I'm driving the car and see a runner I'm tempted to stop and join in – and I'm so pleased to see more females running nowadays. I've now lost 10 pounds and big Sunday lunches are a thing of the past. I feel terrific: full of energy and confidence. I wish I had done all this years ago.

And the most engaging comment, in one of the newsletters the Fun Runners circulated to each other, came from Diana, the typist:

> I used to enjoy typing and I thought it was good exercise. At least I had fit fingers! But I have spent the last half hour typing about other people's running and thinking how much I would rather be out running than in typing. So I'm going to turn the typewriter off now and get my running shoes out!

At the end of the *Fun Runner '82* project Dr Barrie Gunter summarised the results: at the beginning and end of the five months, he asked all participants to complete a 'Cattell 16 Personality Factor Questionnaire'. The personality of the Fun Runners, men and women together, had changed significantly in five ways. Judged by the Cattell test they became more self-confident; more understanding of the needs and problems of others; less apprehensive; better mannered and less aggressive; and more relaxed and composed. Gunter was especially interested to note what had happened to the women:

> I believe that improved aerobic capacity can bring with it a feeling of well-being for the relatively unfit person – especially when he or she compares the way they feel now, with how they felt just a few weeks or months before.

Gunter emphasised that the most substantial shifts in personality occurred among women; for, according to his assessments, they started the project less self-assured, more tense and less emotionally stable than the men.

Given the pressure put on women right from the start of their lives to shrink away from their physical selves, these

234

findings were hardly surprising. Wilhelm Reich has said: 'Every disturbance of the ability fully to experience one's own body damages self-confidence as well as the unity of the bodily feeling. At the same time it creates the need for compensation.'

At school, girls avoid each others' eyes, in the draughty changing-rooms, before and after the games they have to play. The scene is repeated later in life, in the changing-rooms of clothes shops. At school girls are taught that the 'sporty' girl, the female equivalent of the 'jock', is shallow and stupid. No wonder women so often start an exercise programme fearfully and look for excuses to fail or drop out.

What women are accustomed to is the world where chocolates and flowers and jewels are advertised as signs of love; where glossy magazines encourage fantasies of exotic places and exotic men; where less glossy magazines encourage daydreams of romantic passion. These treats are substitutes for joining in our own lives and creating our own drama, activity and excitement. Life is, should be, something we feel physically; experience through our bodies.

And this is what women are now finding out for themselves. In October 1982 Pineapple Dance Studios held a conference on 'The Exercise Boom' in London. Women of all ages from eighteen to over seventy came from all over Britain to take part. Ex-model Jackie Genova, and ex-Olympic athlete Cindy Gilbert, hold aerobics classes for hundreds of women at a time, in London. Jane Fonda's admirable *Workout Book* has been in the British best-seller charts for over a year. In 1983 four magazines mainly aimed at women who want to be healthy and fit, *Health and Fitness, Work-out, Fitness,* and *New Health*, were launched. Early in 1983 *Running* magazine asked for applications from women, to train for the Avon women-only 10 mile race now held every October at Copthall Stadium in north London. The response, for a magazine ninety-three per cent of whose readers are men, was awe-inspiring: 839 women wrote in.

Aerobics, dance-exercise, popmobility; these are not fads confined to the middle-classes of London and other cities. They are, all together, a new movement springing from and drawing encouragement from other and older disciplines.

A new harmony

Thérèse Bertherat is a French body therapist who doubts the value of conventional forms of exercise that amount to drilling the body. She believes that an aerobic dance class run by a woman sounding like a shrill sergeant-major will only confirm a woman's fears that her body is inadequate. In her book *The Body Has Its Reasons*, Madame Bertherat writes:

> It is possible for you to find the keys to your body again, to find your proper vitality, health and autonomy. But how? Certainly not by regarding your body as a necessarily defective machine that encumbers you, as a machine made up of isolated parts, each of which must be entrusted to a specialist whose authority and verdict you blindly accept.

Yoga, too, encourages us to listen to what our bodies can tell us. So do other disciplines from the East, such as aikido and tai chi, and other forms of movement therapy developed in the West, including bioenergetics and the Alexander Technique. Some women will come to prefer vigorous, even exhausting exercise; the temperament of others will lead them into a quieter means to the same end. Barbara Dale, who runs the Body Workshop in London, teaches exercise based on the Mensendieck method. She combines toning and stretching used as 'active meditation' (in her words) with the aerobic exercise that the body needs to become healthy through fitness. She told me:

> I'm very aware that everything is reflected in your body. During the last 100 years we've come to realise that the mind is a tape of everything that's happened to you. People still don't realise that the body is the very same tape.

The aches and illnesses we suffer, the odd ways we have of sitting, standing, walking, are all part of our map, from which, if we are attentive, we can learn more about ourselves. As I kept on running, I also learned something

236

that previously I would have dismissed as silly and perverse. I learned that discomfort and even pain can be valuable experiences that show what the body can bear; and I enjoyed exploring my limits, and finding that they expanded. Exercise that in one week would be uncomfortable, even painful, became easier in weeks to come, and so I wanted to try harder. How can we know who we are unless we know our limits? How can we learn about ourselves without exploring?

It is believed that the left hemisphere of the brain governs our reason and the right our intuition; and that we in the West have allowed ourselves to be dominated by the left half of our brain. All acts of creation require intuition to interplay with reason, and genius is always inspired by guesses that have nothing to do with logic. The free flow of energy that results from exercise seems to come from our intuitive, even psychic side, and the sense of well-being that invariably follows vigorous exercise may very well derive from a harmony between our two sides.

For women – and men – whose lives are packed with work, stress, decisions and conflict, exercise is the balancer, the healer. Barbara Dale also teaches relaxation, and she told me that:

It's not super-fitness that keeps you healthy. That's fine to help you be more efficient but it's just as important to pay attention to relaxation: it's a very important part of fitness, health, and balance in every way. And if you're in good health you're much better able to cope with conflict.

People change and grow when it is required of them. Anyone who doubts the strength and resilience of women should recall what happened in both World Wars, when the women of Europe were needed as a new labour-force. They took over heavy manual labour   welding, ship-building, machine assembly – previously done by men who before the war would have laughed at the idea of a woman doing 'their work'. It was not by chance that women's suffrage in Great Britain followed so soon after the First World War. As Vera Brittain says in her books, women who had worked in field hospitals in France were not prepared to be told that they were too weak and gentle to act as citizens. Even so, the progress of women's independence has been slow and faltering. After the Second World War public attitudes shifted once again when the men came back from fighting. Women were discouraged from working, with propaganda about 'eight-hour orphans'. Hair styles, fashionably short during the war and reflecting the fact that many women had practical work to do, became long, and as soon as dress material was plentiful Dior created the so-called 'New Look' that resurrected the wasp waist and cumbersome skirts.

The changes that are happening now in the USA and with increasing momentum in Europe have more general causes than war. Women nowadays are somewhat less inclined to listen to male voices of authority, whether these be fathers, bosses, priests, doctors or politicians. Women are more inclined than men to feel the futility and horror of a global arms system created by men. Some of the 30,000 women who in December 1982 encircled the Cruise missile base at Greenham Common, near London, said that politicians saw war as a game and nuclear bombs as their toys. The broad-based protest, especially strong among women, against the arms race and the threat of war is part of a general movement among women to make sure that their voices are heard.

Women are brought up to feed and care for others, to give their time, energy and love to supporting the activity of husband, children or boss. Many women feel uneasy, even guilty, at the idea of taking time to look after and nourish themselves. But just as no plant thrives without watering, no body flourishes without tender loving care, which is not always to be reserved for others. Women who take time each day to enjoy themselves in exercise, and also other forms of play, are less prone to self-destructive feelings of resentment and helplessness. People cannot fully love others unless they have self-esteem. Many women, busy with home and children, neglect themselves, not realising that a self-forgetful attitude breeds indifference and even contempt in others. No one ever thanked a wife or mother for saying, 'I did it all for you.' No wonder that so many women end up rejecting their tired, listless bodies, emphasising this dislike with the self-punishment, if not of drugs, then of dieting.

Self-nourishment

It takes some courage for a woman to give herself time for self-nourishment. Any woman accustomed to dieting will at first resist the idea that good health and a reliable and lasting sense of well-being come from balance between our two fuels, food and air, and from plenty of both. It is hard to appreciate, at first, that the foods most often condemned by diet books – bread, potatoes, root vegetables, cereals and pastas – eaten in whole form are indeed the staff of life. New discoveries involve giving up old beliefs, and a woman who has spent five or twenty-five years dieting and in between diets will not find it easy to accept that her dieting was misspent time.

The self-nurturing and self-assertion involved in exercise go beyond good health. As they grow up, girls are discouraged from being competitive and learn to disparage themselves, and to compare themselves unfavourably with others. Many women deny that they are competitive because they have been taught to put themselves down, to feel that in any of life's races they will fail. Exercise encourages a sense of success; a woman does not have to come first in a sport to discover that she can achieve the physical goals she sets herself, then out-do herself. This self-realisation will dissolve the jealousies and frustrations that women so often come to believe are part of everyday life.

Another reason for changing health and well-being through good food and exercise is that women have found out for themselves that diets simply do not work. But millions of women, although they know that diets do not work for them, still believe that they are at fault, that they are weak, inadequate or greedy. This book is offered as a new freedom for all these women. Diets do not work: and it is their fault, not yours.

Through exercise women can become fit and confident, healthy and full of energy, and gain a new self-respect and a new control over themselves and their lives. And by learning to love themselves they will be able to love others better. By enjoying more of the good things of life, women can understand and discover themselves as whole people, strong, able, active, and in harmony with men.

CHAPTER EIGHT

All You Need To Know

> It seems to me that we are still awfully ignorant of some
> basic biological knowledge regarding the nutritive value of
> food and its additives, its effect on the physiological
> activities of the gut, and the general metabolic
> consequences of this action.
> SIR ERNST CHAIN
> *Food Technology in the 1980s, Address to the Royal Society*

> How we need that unity today, that glowing one-ness of
> body, mind and spirit! More than ever, now that the
> modern era of careless indolence and gluttony is so clearly
> ending, we need the tingling aliveness of every limb, the
> connectedness with nature and other people that only a full
> appreciation of embodiment can bring.
> GEORGE LEONARD
> *The Ultimate Athlete*

The thesis of this book can be summed up in thirty points.
The first ten summarise the effect of dieting on the human
body.

1   Diet books assume that the body works at a set
speed; that some people have a fast metabolic rate, others
a slow one, but that the basic rate for each individual
remains the same. All the sums in diet books that tell
dieters how many calories to consume are based on this
assumption. It is wrong. Metabolic rate is not static; it is
dynamic.

2   Diet books state or imply that most if not all weight
lost on a diet is fat. This is not true. The initial big weight

loss advertised by many diet books as evidence of their effectiveness is of water, and of glycogen, a form of glucose stored together with water in the liver and the muscles. Glycogen is the body's immediately available source of energy.

3   The weight lost on a prolonged diet is of lean tissue from the vital organs and muscles, as well as fat. The more severe the diet, the greater the proportion of lean tissue lost. Metabolic rate slows dramatically during a diet because much of the weight lost is of tissue which, unlike fat, is designed to be metabolically active. Hence the slowing down of weight loss, on a diet.

4   The body of a person on a crash diet reacts as if to starvation; the body of a person on a prolonged diet reacts as if to famine. In each case the body will shed active tissue that consumes a lot of energy and as far as possible will protect the relatively inactive tissue making up the store vital at times of starvation or famine. This inactive tissue is, of course, fat.

5   The human body is more complex than that of any other creature and adapts throughout life to circumstances. The body of an active person will adapt to protect and develop muscle that is constantly used. The body of a sedentary person loses muscle as life goes on. The body of a sedentary dieter will tend to shed muscle because it is little used.

6   Glycogen is essential to the functioning of the body and the brain. Loss of glycogen triggers sensations of intense hunger, even if the stomach is full of food. When a diet is ended the body will replace its glycogen store, and water. But the body of a sedentary dieter will tend not to replace all the metabolically active tissue that has been lost on the diet.

7   Constant dieting trains the body to endure diets. It does this by a process of shedding some lean tissue and replacing it with the fat needed at times of starvation and famine. Fat is itself a source of energy and needs less fuel

than the vital organs. The metabolic rate of the dieter tends to drop from one diet to the next, as the body adapts to need less and less food.

8 Loss of glycogen results in listlessness, depression and irritability. Loss of lean tissue, including muscle, results in the body needing less energy from oxygen in the air, as well as less energy from food, and coming into energy balance at a lower and lower level. Constant dieting makes a person feeble and torpid. This is a cumulative process.

9 A fat person may 'eat like a bird' and gain fat, because of a low metabolic rate caused by being fat. A lean person may 'eat like a horse' and stay lean, because of a high metabolic rate caused by being lean. Women need and use less energy than men; and a light yet fat middle-aged woman who diets regularly can gain weight even on a semi-starvation diet.

10 Dieting slows the body down and creates the conditions for gaining fat. Gradually, after one diet has ended, dieters get fatter and fatter on less and less food. Fat weighs less than lean tissue, and it is perfectly possible to lose weight as a result of accumulative diets and nonetheless gain a greater volume, as well as proportion, of fat to lean tissue.

This is why dieting makes you fat. The next ten points summarise why up to half the population of Western countries tends to get fat, with or without dieting.

11 Diet books imply that the basic requirement of the body is energy from food. This is wrong. The body adapts to very different levels of energy balance, according to circumstances. The body's basic requirement from food is not for quantity but for quality. Above all, what the body needs is nourishment. What is wrong with the food we eat is not its quantity but its lack of quality.

12 Foods lose nourishment when processed. People in the West now eat more processed, 'refined', sugar than

243

any other item of food. Processed sugar is dead, or empty, energy. It supplies calories but no protein, starch, fibre or vitamins and only a trace of minerals. 'Junk' foods supply energy but little or no nourishment. Processed sugar is the chief junk food.

13 Deficiency diseases are caused by a gross lack of nutrients. .These diseases have mild forms that are difficult to diagnose, that may take the form of depression, exhaustion, swings of mood, anxiety, period pains, sleeplessness, irritability, irrational or destructive behaviour. One prime cause of such malaise, almost universal in the West, is eating junk food.

14 The body will always defend itself against the threat of illness. The body of a sedentary person who eats an average amount of processed foods and sugar will continue to signal hunger until enough nourishing food has been eaten. The only way for such a person to get enough nourishment from food is to consume too much energy from food.

15 Sedentary people gain weight and fat as a means of staying healthy. Overweight is not normally a cause of illness. But obesity (not itself a disease) is associated with 'Western' diseases, of the alimentary tract (including the stomach and digestive system) and of the cardiovascular system (the heart, lungs and blood vessels). Processed 'junk' food is a cause of obesity.

16 Some people eat much more processed food and sugar than others. People liable to suffer from deficiency states, or the 'junk food syndrome', for this reason include young office workers and housewives, youngsters, students, people living alone, heavy drinkers, anyone with a 'sweet tooth', and anyone who eats only small amounts of fresh food.

17 Dieters are liable to be in a state of acute malnutrition as a result of their dieting, unless they take great care to eat only nourishing food, including food rich in starch and fibre. Most diets specify cutting out such

244

foods, and it is hard to avoid eating processed sugar, which is present in almost every type of manufactured food. Dieting can cause illness.

18   After a diet regime has ended the body will signal acute hunger, as a means of replacing the nutrients of which it has been starved. This is the reason for the raging appetite and compulsive eating many dieters experience and is another reason why the body frustrates the dieter and becomes fatter after the diet. In the West, well-being often depends on being fat.

19   Processed sugar is worse than useless. As well as replacing nutritious food, it drains the body of some vitamins and is a direct cause of various Western diseases. Eating sugar has the paradoxical effect of lowering the level of sugar in the blood. Processed sugar is a direct cause of diabetes, and heart disease, and is addictive. Eating sugar makes you hungry.

20   The body will always seek a level of energy balance at which the amount of nourishing food eaten will be sufficient for its needs. The body of anyone eating relatively small amounts of good food will therefore tend to slow down. Because people in the West eat a lot of food heavy in energy but poor in nourishment, they get heavier and fatter while eating less.

This is why people in the West tend to get fat. The next ten points summarise the means whereby we can lose fat and gain health.

21   A fire may burn bright with a small amount of good fuel and a gentle draught. With a strong draught a fire will burn faster and higher and use much fuel. As with a domestic fire, so with the human body. Human energy balance is between energy from food and energy from oxygen in the air. The more oxygen we breathe, the more food we will burn.

22   Dieting slows the body down, lowering the

245

metabolic rate as the body adjusts to need less food. Exercise of the right type speeds the body up, raising the metabolic rate as the body adjusts to need more oxygen and therefore also more food. The right type of exercise, using more oxygen, is 'aerobic' exercise, sustained at a point just below breathlessness.

23 Aerobic exercise creates a sense of well-being which is the opposite of the junk food syndrome. This is because anyone who exercises regularly will be eating more food and therefore more nourishing food. The body of the aerobically fit person will also develop a hunger for the nourishing foods it needs; whole foods, rich in protein, starch, fibre, vitamins and minerals.

24 Western life has deprived us of the regular exercise and also of the nourishing food that was enjoyed by people who lived well before industrialisation and that is now enjoyed by settled communities who live away from Western influence. As a rule such people do not get fat and do not suffer from Western diseases. We have much to learn from them.

25 A couple of hours of aerobic exercise a week, divided between four sessions, approximates to the work that peasants do as part of their lives. This exercise develops the muscle that uses fat as fuel and also strengthens the cardiovascular system. The result is a loss of fat, a gain of lean tissue, and a greatly reduced risk of Western diseases, including diabetes and heart disease.

26 Grains (including wheat, corn, rice, oats), legumes (peas and beans) and tubers (especially potatoes) are the staple foods of non-Western societies, as they were in the West before industrialisation. These foods are rich in starch, needed by the body and brain for energy, and also rich in protein, fibre, vitamins and minerals. They are truly the 'Staff of Life'.

27 The importance of fibre, contained within whole foods, is that in effect it exercises the alimentary tract. In all respects food rich in fibre has the opposite effects from

processed sugar on the body. Eating whole food of the type that peasants eat is a vital part of an active life, and will lead to a greatly reduced risk of diseases of the cardiovascular system and alimentary tract.

28   Women have been taught to admire an ideal of slenderness, and to believe that dieting is the means to this end. Because dieting is self-defeating it reinforces the sense of defeat women often feel in a world run to suit men, and is damaging to women's mental as well as physical health. Women will gain self-respect by eating good food.

29   Women have also been taught to reject the ideal of strength, energy and competition, as being men's possessions. So women cling to dieting and resist exercise. It is time now for women to gain the freedom of enjoying their own bodies, to resist unreal stereotypes, and to gain energy, fitness and health by means of exercise that promotes a natural beauty.

30   Sedentary people in the West who eat bad food get fat and go on diets that do not work. Dieting is a perversion caused by bad habits that themselves lead to disease. The body is nourished by good food and regenerated by exercise. These are the principal sources of good health. We become fit and healthy by using all our energies.

Further Reading

Here is a list of books and writers for the reader who wants to gain more information.

A recent account of overweight and obesity in Britain, whose recommendations, published as this book was being completed, have greatly encouraged its thesis, is:
Royal College of Physicians of London, *Obesity, Journal of the RCP,* January 1983

This follows an earlier American report of the McGovern Committee:
United States Senate, Select Committee on Nutrition and Human Needs, *Eating in America: Dietary Goals for the United States*, MIT Press, London, 1977

The group of British doctors who established the connection between processed carbohydrate (sugar in particular) and disease, and between unprocessed carbohydrate (rich in protein, starch, fibre, vitamins and minerals) and health, include Sir Robert McCarrison, Surgeon-Captain T L Cleave, Dr Hugh Trowell, Dr Denis Burkitt, Dr A R P Walker and Dr Neil Painter. They are supported by Sir Douglas Black, Sir Francis Avery Jones, Sir Richard Doll and, outstanding among a younger generation, Dr Kenneth Heaton and Professor Philip James. Anything written by these doctors is recommended, in particular:

Denis Burkitt, *Don't Forget Fibre in Your Diet*, Martin Dunitz, London, 1979

T L Cleave, George Campbell and Neil Painter, *Diabetes, Coronary Thrombosis and the Saccharine Disease,* John Wright and Sons, Bristol, 1969

T L Cleave, *The Saccharine Disease*, John Wright and Sons, Bristol, 1974

Sir Robert McCarrison, *Nutrition and Health*, The McCarrison Society, London, 1982

Royal College of Physicians of London, *Medical Aspects of Dietary Fibre*, Pitman Medical, London, 1980

Hugh Trowell, Denis Burkitt and Kenneth Heaton, *Dietary Fibre, Refined Carbohydrate Foods and Disease*, Academic Press, London, 1984

Four textbooks on nutrition, the analysis of food, and on vitamins and minerals, are:

A A Paul and D A T Southgate, *McCance and Widdowson's The Composition of Foods*, HMSO, London, 1978

The Staff of *Prevention* magazine, *The Complete Book of Vitamins*, Rodale Press, Aylesbury, 1978

The Staff of *Prevention* magazine, *The Complete Book of Minerals For Health*, Rodale Press, Aylesbury, 1981

Eleanor Noss Whitney and Eva May Nunnelley Hamilton, *Understanding Nutrition*, West Publishing Co., St Paul, Minneapolis, 1981

Remarkably, there is no good up-to-date book on the relationship between fitness and health, or on the relationship between food, health and disease, originally published in Britain. Doctors and scientists are trained to specialise, and so are uneasy when asked to generalise about people as a whole. Meanwhile, a number of authorities are contributing key research to specialist journals. These include Professor John Durnin and Professor J N Morris, in Britain; Professor Ralph Paffenbarger and Professor Peter Wood, in the USA; and Professor Per-Olof Åstrand and Professor Bengt Saltin, in Scandinavia.

The handbooks of Dr Kenneth Cooper, the pioneer of aerobic exercise, are still valuable and include his own training programmes. These are:

Kenneth Cooper, *The New Aerobics*, Bantam, London, 1970

Kenneth Cooper, *The Aerobics Way*, Corgi, London, 1978

The best book for warm-up exercises, and general advice for the jogger, is:
Bob Glover and Jack Shepherd, *The Runner's Handbook*, Penguin, London, 1982

The jogger who intends to become a long-distance runner and run marathons should ignore the 'expert' training schedules of 60 miles a week. This is far too much. With the readers of *Running* magazine I have devised a schedule for runners who want to keep their health, friends and sanity:
Geoffrey Cannon ('Fun Runner'), 'The 88 + 1 Training Schedule', *Running* magazine, London, January, March, April, 1983

For women who exercise the two outstanding books for theory, history and practice are:
Ken Dyer, *Catching Up The Men: Women and Sport*, Junction Books, London, 1982
Jane Fonda, *Jane Fonda's Workout Book*, Allen Lane, London, 1982

Two classic books on exercise physiology are:
Per-Olof Åstrand and Kaare Rodahl, *Textbook of Work Physiology*, McGraw Hill, Maidenhead, 1978
William McArdle, Frank Katch and Victor Katch, *Exercise Physiology: Energy, Nutrition and Human Performance*, Kimpton, London, 1981

Two books on food and health written by women with people in mind, are outstanding. These are:
Leslie Kenton, *The Joy of Beauty*, Century, London, 1983
Jane Brody's *Nutrition Book*, Bantam, London, 1982

Cook-books are beginning to be published, written by lovers of good food whose recipes are delicious and also healthy. These include:
Richard and Elizabeth Cook, *Sugar Off!*, Great Ouse Press,

Cambridge, 1983
Evelyn Findlater, *Wholefood Cooking*, Frederick Muller, London, 1983
Dr Elizabeth Forsythe, *The High-Fibre Gourmet*, Pelham, London, 1983
Janet Horsley, *Sugar-Free Cookbook*, Prism Press, Dorchester, 1983
Colin Tudge, *Future Cook: A Taste Of Things To Come*, Mitchell Beazley, London, 1980

Three new British magazines, all designed to develop knowledge of health, fitness and food, are:
Fitness (published as a sister magazine to *Running* magazine)
Health and Fitness
New Health (of which I am the editor)
Readers who want to keep up-to-date with new research and ideas are encouraged to read these magazines.

Index

264

DO YOU LIVE ALONE?

Then here's the perfect handbook for you . . .

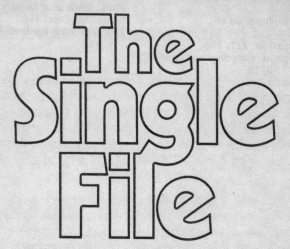

The Single File

DEANNA MACLAREN

Whatever your reason for living alone, THE SINGLE
FILE will prove an invaluable handbook. Packed full
of information and advice on everything from
accommodation to travelling solo; the social scene to
handling money, THE SINGLE FILE is a sensible,
warm and encouraging book that no 'single' can
afford to be without.
Make your single life the *best* time of your life, get
THE SINGLE FILE – on sale now.

REFERENCE   0 7221 5708 8   £1.95

GEORGINA O'HARA
MONEYWOMAN
How to make money work for you

Whether you work for your money or not, you can make money work for you. As anyone who has ever tried to balance their budget knows, there's a world of difference between spending money and using it. MONEYWOMAN shows you how to use it.

MONEYWOMAN shows dozens of different ways in which you can deal with your personal finances, whether you're working or not, married – with or without children – single, divorced, widowed, separated or living with someone.

MONEYWOMAN translates the jargon, shows you the options and lets you choose. It's your money and your life. This book helps you to make the most of both.

REFERENCE   0 7221 6509 9   £1.75

LET YOURSELF BE TEMPTED BY

Forbidden Fruits and Forgotten Vegetables

GEORGE AND NANCY MARCUS

Celery Root, Dandelion, Fennel, Kale, Mango, Okra, Persimmon, Pomegranate, Quince and many more . . . A delicious and unusual variety of once rare and costly fruits and vegetables can now be bought easily and cheaply in this country all the year round. FORBIDDEN FRUITS AND FORGOTTEN VEGETABLES shows you how to cook an appetizing assortment of sensationally different dishes – from North African Lamb Stew with Okra to Jerusalem Artichoke Soufflé and Persimmon Whipped Cream Pie – using innovative and little-known ingredients.

COOKERY   0 7221 5732 0   £2.95

The Book Of
ROYAL
LISTS

CRAIG BROWN & LESLEY CUNLIFFE

What should you serve the Royal Family if they drop in for dinner?
How does the Queen keep her Corgies content?
Which clergyman did Prince Charles throw into the fountain at Balmoral?
What are Princess Diana's favourite sweets?
Which television programmes does the Queen Mother like best?
How can you recognise a Royal racing pigeon?

The Royal Family is no ordinary family, and Royal Lists are not like ordinary lists. Here at last are the answers to all the questions that have intrigued dedicated Royal-watchers, loyal patriots, convinced monarchists and the millions of adoring fans around the world who follow every move of Britain's first family.

THE BOOK OF ROYAL LISTS is the most comprehensive collection of information ever assembled about the British Royal Family and their ancestors. Witty and informed, amusing but respectful, it surprises, charms and dazzles.

HUMOUR   0 7221 1934 8   £2.50

A SELECTION OF BESTSELLERS FROM SPHERE

FICTION

THE MISTS OF AVALON	Marion Bradley	£2.95 ☐
THE INNOCENT DARK	J. S. Forrester	£1.95 ☐
TRUE DETECTIVE	Max Allan Collins	£3.50 ☐
THE ALMIGHTY	Irving Wallace	£1.95 ☐
GREEN HARVEST	Pamela Oldfield	£1.95 ☐

FILM AND TV TIE-INS

THEY CALL ME BOOBER FRAGGLE	Michaela Muntean	£1.50 ☐
RED AND THE PUMPKINS	Jocelyn Stevenson	£1.50 ☐
THE RADISH DAY JUBILEE	Sheilah B. Bruce	£1.50 ☐
MINDER	Anthony Masters	£1.50 ☐
SHROUD FOR A NIGHTINGALE	P. D. James	£1.95 ☐

NON-FICTION

DIETING MAKES YOU FAT	Geoffrey Cannon & Hetty Einzig	£1.95 ☐
EMMA & CO	Sheila Hocken	£1.50 ☐
THE PEAUDOUCE FAMILY WELCOME GUIDE	Malcolm Hamer & Jill Foster	£2.95 ☐
TWINS	Peter Watson	£1.75 ☐
THE FRUIT AND NUT BOOK	Helena Radecka	£6.95 ☐

All Sphere books are available at your local bookshop or newsagent, or can be ordered direct from the publisher. Just tick the titles you want and fill in the form below.

Name _____

Address _____

_____

Write to Sphere Books, Cash Sales Department, P.O. Box 11, Falmouth, Cornwall TR10 9EN

Please enclose a cheque or postal order to the value of the cover price plus:

UK: 45p for the first book, 20p for the second book and 14p for each additional book ordered to a maximum charge of £1.63.

OVERSEAS: 75p for the first book and 21p per copy for each additional book.

BFPO & EIRE: 45p for the first book, 20p for the second book plus 14p per copy for the next 7 books, thereafter 8p per book.

Sphere Books reserve the right to show new retail prices on covers which may differ from those previously advertised in the text or elsewhere, and to increase postal rates in accordance with the PO.